B

The Natural Diabetes Cure

Curing Blood Sugar Disorders Without Drugs

by
Roger Mason

The Natural Diabetes Cure

Curing blood sugar disorders without drugs

The most researched and comprehensive and complete book written on curing blood sugar disorders naturally with diet, supplements, hormones, and exercise.

Roger Mason

The Natural Diabetes Cure
by
Roger Mason

Copyright Winter 2005 by Roger Mason
All Rights Reserved

ISBN 978-1-884820-80-9
Library of Congress Catalog Number 2006900412
Categories: 1. Health 2.
Printed in the U.S.A.
1st Printing Winter 2005

Published by Safe Goods
561 Shunpike Rd.
Sheffield, MA 01257
(413) 229-7935
www.safegoodspub.com

Contents

About This Book

We will treat all blood sugar conditions as basically the same in this book. Metabolic Syndrome, type 1 or 2 diabetes, gestational, insulin resistance, hypoglycemia or any other glucose problem is cured by the same means - diet, proven supplements, natural hormones, exercise, not using prescription drugs, and avoiding bad habits. Unfortunately, fasting cannot be used generally until you are well, although calorie restriction should be.

As long as you have an intact pancreas you can cure yourself if you want to. Even those people whose pancreas has irreversibly atrophied or been surgically removed can dramatically improve their lives and their health and reduce their insulin requirements. There is massive research behind this book, but only a fraction of it is quoted. Everything in here is backed up by voluminous published, international, clinical studies. Unfortunately, every year the researchers of the world more and more choose to study toxic allopathic drugs to treat blood sugar disorders instead of whole foods, natural supplements, balancing the rest of the endocrine system, and exercise.

The answer is not separate from the problem; the answer is always *within* the problem itself. *Diabetes and other blood sugar disorders are caused by what we eat and the way the live.* You can therefore cure yourself by making healthier food choices and living better. Even those who are genetically and racially predisposed to such conditions can cure themselves naturally.

Diabetics often become depressed due to the suffering, the constant glucose monitoring, the incessant medication, the terrible side effects as they age, and knowing they will have a short lifespan of increasingly poor quality. No attempt will be made to deal with this psychology. As you cure yourself your psychological outlook will improve immensely.

Medical professionals will tell you that diabetes and other blood sugar disorders are incurable, and there are no natural solutions. You should be able to heal yourself in one year if you are sincere. Diseases are easy to cure; patients aren't.

Overview

Diabetes is the fastest growing epidemic in the Western world. One in three American children will grow up and needlessly develop diabetes. 24% of American adults are insulin resistant and 45% of adults over the age of 60 are insulin resistant. Two thirds of Americans are overweight and one third are outright obese. Now it is common to see overweight and diabetic children. In the last three decades diabetes and other blood sugar problems have become epidemics in all of the developed countries of the world. It is estimated that about 18 million Americans have diabetes, 16 million are prediabetic, and a whopping 60 million (one in five) have metabolic syndrome. America leads the world in blood sugar dysmetabolism for a very simple reason; we have the greatest affluence as well as the worst diets and lifestyles. We eat twice the calories we need, 42% fat calories (nearly all saturated animal fats), twice the protein we need, and over 160 pounds of various sugars and sweeteners annually we don't need at all. Our food is heavily refined, chemicalized, and preserved. *We are overfed and undernourished.* America is the fattest country in the world and few us get any regular exercise.

The obvious causes of diabetes are our diet and lifestyle. Therefore, changing our diet and lifestyle will both prevent and cure blood sugar disorders. You must be willing to change your life if you want to get well. The medical profession cannot help you; you must help yourself. Doctors and clinics just cannot do anything for you. You have to be your own doctor and your own savior. You must be willing to eat better foods, get regular exercise, and change your lifestyle

Please read my book *Zen Macrobiotics for Americans* to learn more about eating whole natural foods. *The Natural Diabetes Cure* is the most researched, effective, documented, comprehensive and complete book on diabetes and blood sugar problems available.

Chapter 1: About Diabetes

The fastest growing disease in the world! The Metabolic Syndrome, or pre-diabetes is the fastest rising epidemic on the planet. This condition is characterized by:

OBESITY
INSULIN RESISTANCE
DYSLIPIDEMIA
HYPERTENSION
HIGH INSULIN

Obesity may be responsible for 75% of the problem. Insulin resistance most often goes undiagnosed. Hypertension is another epidemic and 75% of such people have diabetes. High blood cholesterol, and especially triglycerides, are normal. High blood insulin levels also go undiagnosed. Almost one in four American adults suffer from Metabolic Syndrome and will soon be diagnosed with diabetes. According to the Center for Disease Control (CDC) in Atlanta one in three children born today in the United States will develop type 2 diabetes. *One in three American children will be diabetic!* Age is one of the biggest factors since one in five Americans over the age of 65 is diabetic. Stress is also an important factor, and most Westerners are under a good deal of self imposed stress. No other country in the world will approach these statistics. Blacks, Latins, Asians, and Amerindians suffer disproportionately. American Pima Indians, for example, have an almost 50% rate of outright diabetes. Mexican Pima Indians, on the other hand, who follow their traditional diet and lifestyle, have a very low rate of just a few percent. One fourth of adult Navajo Indians are diabetic according to CDC statistics. Asian adults in America generally have almost a 40% rate of diabetes, yet this is rare in the rural areas of Asia. Many Asian cities have now largely adopted the Western high fat, high sugar, refined foods diet and their diabetes rates are soaring. Latin adults in America generally have a 15% diabetes rate but not in their native countries. In Papua

New Guinea - possibly the least civilized country in the world - diabetes is basically unknown. Black American adults now have about a 10% diabetes rate, yet this is rare in Africa where they eat their traditional diet. Caucasian American adults have the lowest rate of about 5%.

We are only going to discuss blood sugar metabolism in general rather than the metabolic syndrome, type 1, type 2, gestational, hypoglycemia, insulin resistance and other conditions. These are all simply facets of the same basic problem. Diabetes is the most serious and deadly condition. Currently this is the fifth leading cause of death in the U.S. and will soon be the fourth leading cause. Almost twenty million Americans now have actual diabetes, which means about one in every fifteen. In addition there are probably about six million more, mostly poor people, who have diabetes and simply haven't been medically diagnosed. A million more are newly diagnosed every year. These are mostly the impoverished and elderly who can't afford the medical care they need. All in all, this would mean about one in twelve Americans are diabetic, with the rates rising every year! This is the fastest growing disease of all worldwide plain and simple. India and China are also coping with growing epidemics. In the 1990s the diabetes rate in America increased a full one third. Almost $150 billion a year is spent directly and indirectly worldwide on diabetes treatment. This money is basically wasted on toxic, harmful prescription drugs such as acarbose, metformin, and sulfonylureas that temporarily cover up some of the symptoms of the problem. (Rezulin was taken off the market due to the extreme side effects.) None of these drug therapies are effective.

The situation gets worse when you consider metabolic syndrome or Syndrome X. The CDC recently studied 8,814 men and women. They found that 22% of them exhibited at least three of the six factors of metabolic syndrome. People over 60 with three of the factors had a 44% rate, or double the average. This means almost half of Americans over the age of 60 are pre-diabetic. This condition is called "pre-diabetes" since such people can plan on

8

becoming diabetic within ten years.

Again, the basic indications are obesity (especially abdom-inal), insulin resistance, elevated blood sugar, high cholesterol and triglycerides, and hypertension. There are three main types of diabetes. Type 1 (insulin dependent) is due to the inability of the beta cells in the pancreas to produce insulin. Only 5% to 10% of people suffer from type 1. Surprisingly Caucasians are more susceptible to this form. This usually happens in childhood or adolescence. These patients have to inject insulin since they can't produce it naturally. If the pancreas has been removed or is atrophied the condition cannot be cured. Quality of life can be improved immensely and insulin requirements can be reduced dramatically by following the advice in this book. Pancreas transplants just don't work unfortunately. Transplanting a pancreas from a cadaver to a type 1 diabetic requires dangerous anti-rejection drugs and there are countless problems. Transplants of just the pancreatic beta cells also promises much more than is delivered. Within twenty years science should be able to successfully perform this procedure, but that will merely be allopathic.

Type 2 diabetics (non-insulin dependent) produce insulin, but the cells simply don't react well to it anymore. This type is very curable (usually in one year) as the pancreas not only produces insulin, but usually overproduces it since the effectiveness is so reduced. The third type is called "gestational diabetes" since it only effects pregnant women. For some reason, pregnant women are more susceptible to diabetes than anyone else.

The best way to understand the dysfunction of insulin and blood sugar is the theory of *oxidative stress*. Here free radicals run rampant through the body and use up our antioxidants - glutathione, SOD (superoxide dismutase), beta carotene, vitamin E, vitamin C, CoQ10, melatonin, lipoic acid, and others. This is why it is so important to, first of all, lower the oxidative stress with better diet and exercise. Secondly, we need to take all the known

9

antioxidant supplements to neutralize the excess free radicals. These supplements are discussed in detail in chapters six and seven. The high rates of alcohol and nicotine use add to oxidative stress. Surprisingly, while coffee worsens oxidative stress and has very serious health effects, it doesn't seem to worsen blood sugar metabolism. The scientists of the world are in basic agreement that free radical oxidative stress is central to blood sugar conditions.

About a half million Americans die every year from diabetes. If you are diabetic you have about three times the rate of strokes, about three times the rate of heart attacks, and greatly increased atherosclerosis (clogged arteries) in most patients. Remember that heart disease is the number one cause of death and the biggest killer by far. Blindness and vision problems are called "diabetic retinopathy" and are epidemic for people with impaired blood sugar metabolism. Amputation of limbs due to poor circulation is common. Various cancers, gastrointestinal infections, osteoporosis, erectile dysfunction, poorly healing wounds, kidney infections and failure, are all part and parcel here, the pancreas deteriorates, nerve damage of various kinds can be expected, liver disease is routine, and skin infections (especially Staphylococcus) are routine. The list of side effects is almost endless since the total health of the body is destroyed.

If you have type 1 diabetes pancreas transplants and beta cell (the insulin producing pancreatic cells) transplants just don't work well at all. Dangerous anti-rejection drugs are required for one thing. You can improve your health immensely with the information in this book and reduce your medication. Even if your pancreas has been removed or atrophied beyond repair, you can still live a good life with minimal oral insulin. Anyone with type 2 diabetes can cure themselves within a year and live a normal, healthy life.

Chapter 2: Diagnosis

What are the diagnostic indications of the blood sugar dysmetabolism? Look for any combination of obesity, hypertension, insulin resistance, low HDL cholesterol, high LDL cholesterol, high triglycerides, hypertension, elevated uric acid, high C-reactive protein, hypercoagulability of the blood, fasting blood glucose over 85 (not merely under 100), low white blood cell count and proteinuria (protein in the urine). Age is critical here; the older you are the more blood sugar problems you can expect to have. Diabetes rates go up dramatically after the age of 50. Genetics is obviously important and any family history of such problems increases your chances. Obesity is one of the cornerstone factors and an entire chapter is devoted to this. Race is very important, so you are far more at risk if you are of African, Asian, Amerindian, or Latin origin. Caucasians have the lowest rates (except type 1). Smokers get far more diabetes than others, as do people who drink substantial amounts of alcohol. If you are a woman with polycystic ovary syndrome (PCOS) you can almost count on having insulin resistance (an inexpensive sonogram will diagnose PCOS).

What specific diagnostic tests can you get? When you get your standard, basic blood analysis profile you'll test glucose, uric acid, white blood cell count, total cholesterol, blood coagulation, HDL (high density or "good"), LDL (low density or "bad"), and triglycerides. Total cholesterol should be about 150 ideally and very definitely well under 200. Triglycerides are very crucial here and should be under 100. Uric acid and white blood cell count should be in normal range. Request CRP and proteinuria tests to go with these. Surprisingly, you do not need to get your insulin tested. You should also have your homocysteine tested if you are over 40 as a predictor of coronary heart disease (CHD), but it won't help diagnose diabetes. Homocysteine will accurately predict insulin resistance and the side effects of diabetes such as neuropathy and retinopathy, however. Currently we do not have accurate tests to

11

determine total oxidative stress or general free radical levels. It is costly and unnecessary to test the basic status of antioxidants such as SOD, glutathione, vitamin C, beta carotene and vitamin E. The antioxidant supplements you should take are discussed in great detail in *Chapter 6: Supplements.*

Blood pressure is basic here and you should look for a reading of 120/80 or better. In 2006 my ninth book *Lower Blood Pressure Without Drugs* will be published explaining how to normalize your blood pressure naturally. Following the advice in this book you can have healthy blood pressure levels within 90 days. Inexpensive home electronic monitors are widely available.

The most important test you can get is a glucose tolerance test (GTT). This is more predictive than testing your insulin level per se as it shows the metabolism and sensitivity of your insulin. If your blood sugar level is over 85 you need to do this. A GTT is the "gold standard", accurate, well known, inexpensive, but very underutilized. It is just not commonly done due to lack of knowledge in the medical profession. Simply get a one hour, one blood draw test (you should already know your fasting blood glucose level so you won't need a draw before you drink the glucose solution). You go to the doctor in the morning having not eaten for at least 12 hours. You'll drink a 75g cup of glucose solution and wait one hour. Your blood glucose will then be tested to determine the effectiveness of your insulin response. This tells you far more than simply measuring fasting insulin levels per se.

You can do your own GTT test at home without a doctor if you want. Buy some glucose on the Internet and weigh out 75 grams (basically two and a half ounces) on a postal or other scale. Buy an electronic glucose meter at the drug store. The companies are literally giving these away for free so you'll buy their very costly test strips. Test your fasting glucose level, drink the glucose solution, wait one hour, and test your glucose again.

There are exotic tests you can get such as malondialdehyde,

thrombomodulin, adoponectin, leptin, plasminogen, tumor necrosis factor-alpha (TNF), fibrinogen and others. These are simply not practical or necessary, plus they can be expensive and hard to obtain. It is very difficult to test the amount of oxidative stress you suffer from or your antioxidant status in general. There just isn't any reason to spend the time and money on these tests because the ones we'll talk about tell us more than enough. Your attention needs to be on curing yourself and changing your diet and lifestyle rather than getting exotic diagnostic tests you don't need.

Generally people can simply get their total cholesterol (TC) and triglycerides (TG) tested. Here you also need to test your high density ("good") HDL and your low density ("bad") LDL levels. Your TC should ideally be 150 mg/dl. The media and medical profession will tell you that a 200 level or less is good, but that's just not the case at all. Even if you have genetically high cholesterol you can still keep your level well under 200 with diet, supplements, hormones and exercise. Please read my book *Lower Cholesterol Without Drugs*. *The TG level is the most important blood lipid marker* of all for blood sugar problems. Even vegetarians can have high levels due to an inordinate intake of sweets. Your TG means more than your TC, LDL or HDL. You should keep your triglyceride level below 100. You can do this with the same means as for total cholesterol. People with blood sugar problems usually have low HDL and high LDL levels. You can raise your HDL and lower your LDL the same way.

Fasting blood plasma glucose is part of your basic routine blood analysis. Your level should be at 85 mg/dl or less. Levels of 100 and higher are clearly pre-diabetic. You need to have low blood sugar, and the usual accepted level of 100 and less just isn't good enough. Doctors will tell you that any reading under 100 is "normal", but this isn't true. This was proven at the Rikshospitalet Hospital in Norway with a 22 year follow-up study of 1,998 healthy men. The men with glucose levels of 85 or less lived the longest and had the least cardiovascular disease - the biggest killer of men and women in the world by far.

C-reactive protein (CRP) is a marker for inflammation and a very important test for CHD conditions. The best study on this came from the Quebec Heart Institute. CRP correlates with obesity, blood glucose impairment, insulin resistance, hypertension, triglycerides, and uric acid. It has been found the CRP also accurately predicts blood sugar disorders. CRP is positively associated with obesity, impaired glucose function, the metabolic syndrome generally, and outright type 2 diabetes in otherwise healthy people. Everyone over the age of 40 should annually get a CRP test with their regular yearly checkup and blood analysis. Even children and young people can benefit from a CRP test.

Uric acid is part of a standard blood analysis. High uric acid is clearly associated with type 2 diabetes and the metabolic syndrome in general. Surprisingly, low uric acid can be associated with type 1 diabetes. This is not due to better diets in people with type 1, but rather excessive excretion of uric acid in this condition. High uric acid levels are associated with obesity, high triglycerides, high systolic blood pressure, and a high total cholesterol to low HDL ratio. High uric acid comes from breakdown of purines and from eating meat and other animal products which contain purines. While purines are found in most all foods, vegetarians and people who eat seafood do not get this condition. High uric acid is found in wealthy developed countries basically.

There should be very low levels of albumin (protein) in your urine. You can use urine test strips from the drug store instead of a urine analysis from a physician. This is one very good indication of kidney health. Eating a low protein diet (Americans eat twice the protein they need which causes many health problems) will quickly cure this.

Again, don't get carried away with diagnostic tests. What we've discussed here is beyond what you really need. Put your energy and attention into curing yourself.

Chapter 3: Whole Grains: The Staff of Life

Whole grains are literally "the staff of life," and have been the staple food of almost all civilizations throughout history. Since man started agriculture about 10,000 years ago, whole grains have been the principal food of most all people in the world. This emancipated us from being mere primitive hunters and gatherers. Whole grains should be the very basis of your diet.

The real cure for blood sugar dysfunction of any kind is making better food choices and eating whole natural foods. *Diet is everything!* Eating fat, sugars, refined foods, and just plain too much food is the basic cause of blood sugar problems. Eating whole, natural, high-fiber, low-fat, low-sugar foods is the cure. Supplements, hormones, and exercise are secondary to what you eat. You can cure diabetes and other conditions with diet alone, but that is difficult, takes longer, and is simply not necessary. Traditional Japanese macrobiotics has a very limited selection of foods, and does not use supplements, natural hormones, or even fasting. Please read my book *Zen Macrobiotics for Americans* to learn more about making the best food choices, proven supplements, hormone balance, and sensible fasting.

Our grains are refined, and we eat white rice, white bread, white pasta and white flour. The ideal diet is based on whole grains, beans, green and yellow vegetables, local fruit, seafood (vegetarians can drop this), soups and salads. That means no more red meat, poultry, eggs, dairy products, refined foods, nightshade vegetables (potatoes, tomatoes, peppers, and eggplants), or tropical foods such as citrus, bananas and mangoes.

Whole grains such as wheat, rice, barley, corn, rye, oats, buckwheat, spelt, and millet should be the basis of your diet. Beans of all types should also be a staple. This is very easy to do by eating such foods as whole grain pasta, whole grain breads, brown rice, oatmeal, steamed barley, whole grain breakfast cereals,

15

polenta, and unrefined grain products.

At the University of Minnesota (Proceedings of the Nutrition Society v. 62, 2003) "Epidemiological Support For the Protection of Whole Grains Against Diabetes" was published. This impressive review was based on 160,000 men and women. "There is accumulating evidence to support the hypothesis that whole-grain consumption is associated with a reduced risk of incident type 2 diabetes. It may also improve glucose control in diabetic individuals." They went on further to say, "Observations in non-diabetic individuals support an inverse relationship between whole-grain consumption and fasting insulin levels." The more whole grains you eat the more effective your insulin is metabolized in other words. "Glucose control improved with diets rich in whole grain in feeding studies of subjects with type 2 diabetes."

At the National Public Health Institute in Finland (American Journal of Clinical Nutrition v. 77, 2003) "Whole-grain Fiber Intake and the Incidence of Type 2 Diabetes" was published. 2,286 men and 2,030 women were studied. "An inverse association between whole-grain intake and the risk of type 2 diabetes was found." The more whole grains people eat the less diabetes they suffer from in countries all over the world.

At Yonsei University in Korea (Atherosclerosis, Thrombosis & Vascular Biology v. 21, 2001) men were fed whole grain based diets for only 16 weeks. In that short time their blood glucose fell a full 24% and their insulin levels fell 14%. It was also found that plasma lipid peroxidation fell 28% which lowered the risk for coronary heart illnesses. All this in only four months! Imagine what would happen if you made whole grains a staple for the rest of your life.

In a collective study between the USDA, Harvard, Tufts and other institutions (American Journal of Clinical Nutrition v. 76, 2002) one of the famous Framingham series of studies was used to study whole grain intake for the prevention of type 2

16

diabetes. The Framingham studies have been the longest, most complete, and comprehensive of any human health research ever performed. "After adjustment for potential confounding factors, whole-grain intake was inversely associated with body mass index, waist-to-hip ratio, total cholesterol, LDL cholesterol, and fasting insulin." This means the more whole grains you eat the slimmer you'll be, your blood sugar and insulin will be normal, and the lower your cholesterol will be. They said further, "The inverse association between whole-grain intake and fasting insulin was most striking among overweight participants." Their conclusion was, "Increased intake of whole grains may reduce disease risk by means of favorable effects on metabolic risk factors."

At the famous Harvard University (American Journal of Clinical Nutrition v. 75, 2002) "Whole Grain May Reduce Risk of Type 2 Diabetes" was published. "Insulin sensitivity may be an important mechanism whereby whole-grain foods reduce the risk of type 2 diabetes and heart disease." They suggested, "People should be encouraged to replace the refined-grain foods in their diet, such as white bread and bagels, refined-grain breakfast cereals and white rice with whole grain choices." The researchers found that insulin sensitivity improved in a group of overweight and obese adults when they ate a diet rich in whole-grain foods such as brown rice, oats, barley, and corn. The conclusion was, "Whole-grain foods may have favorable effects on insulin sensitivity. These effects may reduce the risk of type 2 diabetes and heart disease." It really is easy to replace refined grain foods with whole grains. They taste much better and have more flavor.

Also from Harvard Medical School et al (American Journal of Clinical Nutrition v. 76, 2002) "Whole-Grain Intake and Risk of Type 2 Diabetes". Over 50,000 men we followed for 12 years as part of the Health Professionals Study. The men who ate the most whole-grain foods had the least diabetes, while the men who ate the least whole-grain foods had the most diabetes. Their conclusion was clear, "A diet high in whole grains is associated with a reduced risk of type 2 diabetes. Efforts should be made to replace refined-grain with whole-grain foods." Over 50,000 men proved this at Harvard and there were other published studies here that clinically proved eating whole grains prevent and cure blood sugar conditions.

At the University of Minnesota this same phenomenon was found with women (American Journal of Clinical Nutrition v. 71, 2000). 36,000 women were studied for six years. The more whole grains they ate the less diabetes they suffered from. "These data support a protective role for whole grains, cereal fiber, and dietary magnesium in the development of diabetes in older women." They found that, "Total grain, whole-grain, total dietary fiber, and dietary magnesium intakes showed strong inverse correlations with incidence of diabetes after adjustment for potential nondietary confounding variables." The more whole grains the less diabetes.

Neal Barnard at the Physicians Committee for Responsible Medicine (PCRM) published a study "Type 2 Diabetes and the Vegetarian Diet" (American Journal of Clinical Nutrition v. 78, 2004). Neal and the PCRM are doctors who honestly believe in natural health. "Long-term cohort studies have indicated that whole-grain consumption reduces the risk of both type 2 diabetes and cardiovascular disease. The use of whole-grain or traditionally processed cereals and legumes has been associated with improved glycemic control in both diabetic and insulin-resistant individuals." This is from a group of prominent medical doctors.

Our own government verifies this at the USDA Human Nutrition Research Center in MD (Journal of the American College of Nutrition v. 19, 2000). "Consumption of (whole) grains has been reported to control or improve glucose tolerance and reduce insulin resistance. There are a number of mechanisms by which (whole) grains may improve glucose metabolism and delay or prevent the progression of impaired glucose tolerance to insulin resistance and diabetes. A number of whole grain foods and grain fiber sources are beneficial in reducing insulin resistance and improvement in glucose tolerance." They strongly suggest eating more servings of whole grain foods every day.

Doctors at the Inter-Medic Medical Group in FL (American Journal of Clinical Nutrition v. 79, 2004) published "Increased Consumption of Refined Carbohydrates and the Epidemic of Type 2 Diabetes in the United States; an Ecologic Assessment." They concluded, "Increasing intakes of refined carbohydrate concomitant with decreasing intakes of fiber paralleled the upward trend in the prevalence of type 2 diabetes observed in the U.S during the 20th century." They point out the extreme change in dietary habits especially in the last 20 years where refined grains, and especially various sweeteners, have become staples now. Consumption of fats, protein, and calories per se has also increased dramatically leading to the current epidemic of diabetes. Eating more whole grains and fewer sweeteners will drastically reduce this problem.

Nathan Pritikin was a real pioneer regarding natural health back in the 1980s. He published two articles (Diabetes Care v. 5, 1982 and v. 6, 1983) on diabetes, diet and exercise. Diabetics on oral medication got off the drugs in just 26 days! by simply eating a whole grain based natural diet and walking everyday. *In less than a month they were drug free!* This is nothing less than amazing and it happened almost a quarter century ago. The supplements we have today were not available at that time generally, nor were natural hormones like melatonin and DHEA. Eating better food and taking a daily walk got most all of them off medication in less than a month. Imagine the results Nathan could get today with proven supplements and natural hormones added to his regimen.

Beans and legumes are very closely related to whole grains, and the benefits of eating them are basically the same. Beans are high in protein, minerals, lignans, and sterols, but low in fat and calories. A four ounce serving of pinto beans, for example, has a mere 117 calories and 1% fat calories. Be sure to include beans and legumes in your daily fare. When you learn to cook beans and make such things as stews, soup, dips and spreads you'll come to enjoy them very much. At Sun-Yat-sen University in China (Ying.

Xuebao v. 20, 1998) diabetics were fed legumes which lowered their glucose levels as well as their C-peptide levels (a basic marker for heart disease). Tofu, by the way, is a heavily refined product lacking in nutrition and only to be used occasionally.

Fiber is one of the important factors here. Whole grains and beans (legumes) have more soluble and insoluble fiber than any other food groups. Meat, poultry, eggs, and dairy products are completely lacking in fiber. There are many studies showing the importance of fiber not only for blood sugar conditions, but for all major diseases. The best way to get fiber is by eating whole grains and beans every day. There are many studies to show that merely the addition of fiber to the diet improves glucose and insulin metabolism dramatically. Fiber supplements are obviously not the answer at all. Eating whole foods gives you plenty of fiber especially whole grains, beans, vegetables and fruits. Americans are generally very fiber deficient from eating refined foods and too many fiber-less animal products.

At Christian-Albrechts University in Germany (Ernaehrung & Medizin v. 17, 2002) the researchers said, "It is not questioned that a diet high in fiber from natural sources consisting of whole grain products, vegetables and fruits may provide greater advantages in diabetic control and in addition will have desirable effects far above of fiber as such."

Mexicans generally have low rates of diabetes largely due to their staples of corn and beans. When they migrate to America and adopt the high fat, high sugar, low fiber diet we eat here they get even higher levels than Caucasians. At the University of Baja (Nutrition Research v. 24, 2004) a crossover study was done where diabetics were fed traditional Mexican foods. In only three weeks very impressive results were obtained especially for dyslipidemia.

Make whole grains and beans your staple foods.

Chapter 4: Fats and Oils

Americans eat about 42% of their calories as saturated, artery clogging, animal fats You only need about 8% unsaturated vegetable oils, so this is more than 500% of what you need, as well as the wrong kind of fats. This is a major reason we lead the world in heart disease, various cancers, diabetes, and other major illnesses.

How do we know for a fact that high fat diets cause diabetes and other blood sugar conditions? Science has shown the countries like China, Viet Nam, Thailand, Korea and Japan have far less diabetes rates. Migration studies have shown that when these people move to the U.S. and adopt the typical Western diet, they get as much and usually *more* blood sugar conditions than other Americans. Studies of what people eat also prove the more fats they consume the more diabetes they get. When diabetics are given low fat diets they improve dramatically. Lastly, studies of the free fatty acids (FFAs) in our blood give irrefutable proof that fats, especially saturated fats, cause blood sugar dysfunction.

We must discuss obesity in relation to fat intake. It is not food that makes you fat; *it is fat that makes you fat.* You simply cannot be overweight or stay overweight if you take dairy products, meat, poultry, and eggs out of your life. Overweight people always eat more fat and have much higher levels of free fatty acids in their blood. These fatty acids are mostly those from animal foods and not those from vegetable sources.

It is not just the saturated fats that cause problems, but also excess vegetable oils due to the omega-6 content. We eat far too many omega-6 fatty acids and far too few omega-3s. This is why flax oil is recommended as a supplement since it is *the* best source of omega-3 fatty acids known. Yes, the Mediterranean diet is better than the Western European and American diets but is *not* the answer at all. Olive oil (monosaturated fats) is not "good for you,"

21

no matter what you read somewhere. Vegetable oils are merely less harmful than animal fats. The point here is to eat a diet of less than 20% total fat - a 30% fat diet is not "low." There is also the problem of hydrogenated and partially hydrogenated "trans fatty acids". These are made by forcing hydrogen gas into vegetable oil under extreme pressure in order to "saturate" the molecule and give the oil longer shelf life. Hydrogenated fats are the worst possible choice and you should avoid them. Read your labels.

The published research in just the last few years on the effect of dietary fats is far too volumous to even attempt to cover. We certainly can mention a few representative studies to prove this very clearly.

There is no doubt excess dietary fat, especially saturated animal fat is one of the basic causes of diabetes. At the University of Athens (Diabetes Care v. 26, 2003) in Greece type 2 diabetics were compared to healthy controls. Their dietary habits were carefully recorded. The ones who ate an average of 30% total fat (with almost half animal fat) had the most diabetes. Please remember the average American eating a whopping 42% total fat and most all of this is animal fat. The doctors concluded, "increased animal fat in the diet may contribute to increased risk of diabetes."

This same phenomenon was demonstrated at the University of Minnesota (American Journal of Clinical Nutrition v. 78, 2003). Almost 3000 adults over 45 had the fatty acids in their blood plasma measured. This is an even better means to determine fat intake than dietary analysis. "Our findings suggest that the dietary fat profile, particularly that of saturated fat, may contribute to the etiology of diabetes." They further said, "...diabetes incidence was significantly and positively associated with the proportion of total saturated fatty acids in plasma.." They specifically found high levels of saturated (animal) fatty acids such as palmitic, palmitoleic and stearic in their serum.

The Women's Health Study (Diabetes Care v. 27, 2004) has been one of the largest and longest ongoing studies of female health involving more than 37,000 women over the age of 45. The amount of red meat they consumed was compared to their incidence of diabetes. "Our data indicate that higher consumption of total red meat, especially processed meats, may increase risk of developing type 2 diabetes in women." They also found that consumption of cholesterol, animal protein, and iron (from animal, not vegetable sources) was also significantly associated with high diabetes rates. Please remember that cholesterol is only found in animal foods and not any plant foods.

We can further prove the relation of fat intake to blood sugar dysmetabolism by studies where people change from high fat to low fat diets, especially with regard to vegetable oils instead of animal fats. At the University of Otago in New Zealand (British Journal of Nutrition v. 83 Supp, 2000) a heavily referenced review of the literature in this area was published. "Lifestyle changes can reduce the progression of impaired glucose tolerance in type 2 diabetes. Insulin sensitivity is enhanced by a range of diet-related changes including reduction of visceral adiposity, and a reduction in saturated fatty acids." Saturated fat intake causes diabetes.

Another heavily referenced review from the University of Uppsala in Sweden in the same journal found high levels of palmitic and palmitoleic fatty acids in the blood serum of diabetics. Similar studies show significant relationships between serum lipid fatty acid composition, which mirrors the quality of the fatty acids in the diet, and insulin sensitivity. You are just not going to have high levels of palmitic, palmoleic and stearic acids in your blood when you eat whole grains, vegetables, fruits and seafood as your basic sustenance as these are basically saturated animal fats.

More proof came from a five year study at the University of Auckland (Diabetes Care v. 24, 2001). Feeding diabetics and controls a low fat diet lowered their blood glucose levels and improved the results for insulin sensitivity on a two hour GTT test.

"Glucose tolerance also improved in patients on the decreased-fat diet". Further, "Thus, the natural history of people at high risk of developing type 2 diabetes is body weight gain and deterioration of glucose tolerance. This process may be ameliorated through adherence to decreased dietary fat intake." They also lost weight by eating as much as they wanted and not increasing their exercise.

The Japanese live longer than any other nationality especially on the island of Okinawa. The urban Japanese have increasingly turned to Western foods, and their health has deteriorated in direct proportion to this. They still have one of the lowest rates of diabetes in the world along with the Chinese, Thai and Viet Namese. At the International Medical Center in Japan (Diabetes Research v. 46, 1999) blood fatty acids of diabetics and healthy controls were studied. The diabetics clearly had higher omega-6 and lower omega-3 fatty acid profiles. The Japanese do eat quite a bit of seafood (containing omega-3s), but very little dairy products, red meat, poultry, and eggs. Eating more seafood was clearly associated with better health and less diabetes.

The famous Temple University in Philadelphia published three studies on free fatty acids in the blood and diabetes (Frontiers in Bioscience v. 3, 1998, Current Opinion in Clinical Nutrition v. 5, 2002, and European Journal of Clinical Nutrition v. 32 Supp, 2002). "Free fatty acids have emerged as a major link between obesity and insulin resistance/type 2 diabetes mellitus." They suggested, "Lowering FFAs in these patients could be a new and promising approach to treat type 2 diabetes."

The literature is replete with studies such as these and the scientific community is in good agreement that high fat diets are one of the major causes of the growing epidemic of type 2 diabetes and other blood sugar problems. We won't quote more. Remember that "low fat" means 20% or less and mostly all unsaturated vegetable oils. This is very easy to do by simply taking animal products out of your diet and eating moderate amounts of seafood.

Chapter 5: Diet, Diet, Diet

It has been repeated over and over that diet and exercise are the way to cure blood sugar conditions of all kinds. Americans eat 42% fat calories (nearly all saturated animal fats), which is five times what they need, twice the protein they need, twice the calories they need, and 160 pounds of various sugars they don't need at all. *We are overfed and undernourished.* This chapter will cover the basic points in my book *Zen Macrobiotics for Americans.* Please read this book to really understand making the best food choices. Please do not be put off by the word "macrobiotics", as it simply means an overall (macro) view of life (bios). You will be eating common foods you grew up with.

One of the basic causes of blood sugar dysmetabolism is a diet high in saturated animal fats. This is documented in the previous chapter. Americans eat over 500% of the fats they need and nearly all of these are saturated animal fats instead of vegetable oils. You do not have to be a vegetarian to cure diabetes and similar illnesses, as you can eat 10% seafood. Ideally you would eat no beef, pork, lamb, poultry, or eggs. Technically, diabetics could eat, say, three 4 ounce portions of lean meat every week and still cure themselves, but this would slow down your progress. The best way to cure yourself is to stop eating red meat, poultry, eggs, and all dairy products - even low fat dairy products.

Milk and milk products are the most allergic foods known for the simple reason they contain lactose (milk sugar). *All adults of all races are lactose intolerant* since they no longer produce the enzyme lactase. Without lactase you simply cannot digest lactose. Everyone over the age of three years old is allergic to dairy products. Fact. Nature provided cow milk for calves and goat milk for baby goats. Lactose-reduced milk is just not the answer here at all, nor are lactase tablets like Lactaid®. Dairy cheese is low in lactose, but is extremely high in saturated animal fat and is a poor food choice. You can use soy, rice, almond or oat milks instead of dairy milk. Very good meltable non-dairy cheeses are available at any grocery store. You can even buy soy cream cheese. Dairy yogurt has twice the amount of milk sugar since powdered milk is added to thicken it. Unfortunately, the current soy yogurts are so full of sugar they are not healthy. Soy ice cream is readily available but, again, is full of sugar.

The studies proving dairy products cause diabetes are numerous. At the Health Protection Branch in Canada (American Journal of Clinical Nutrition v. 51, 1995) they said, "There is a significant positive correlation between consumption of milk protein and incidence of IDDM in data from various countries." They also found that babies who were naturally breast fed were protected from type 1 diabetes. At the A2 Corporation in New Zealand (Medical Hypotheses v. 56, 2001) the researchers clearly found milk proteins related to diabetes, heart disease and outright mortality. "Milk casein consumption also correlates strongly with type 1 diabetes incidence." At the University of Helsinki in Finland (Experimental and Clinical Endocrinology & Diabetes v. 105, 1997), the research showed clearly that milk consumption both for mothers and children is a major cause of type 1 diabetes. Again, at the University of Helsinki (Diabetologia v. 41, 1998) they found the children most allergic to dairy products (based on blood antibodies) had the highest rates of diabetes. At the University of Tampere in Finland (Diabetes v. 49, 2000) they said, "In conclusion, our results provide support for the hypothesis that high consumption of cow's milk during childhood can be diabetogenic." At NIZO Research in the Netherlands (Nahrung v. 43, 1999) the same results were found. At the School of Medicine in Auckland, New Zealand (Diabetologica v. 42, 1999) it was clear that consumption of dairy products were strongly correlated with type 1 diabetes. The research is clear on this: take dairy products completely out of your life. Milk is not good food.

Beans are an excellent food and are very similar to whole grains in their nutritional profile. They are discussed in *Chapter 3: Whole Grains*. There are many delicious varieties of beans

26

available especially in ethnic grocery stores. Beans, bean soups, and bean dips should be a central part of your daily fare. Get a good cookbook and learn how to make more gourmet bean dishes. If you have problems with gas or bloating this is not due to the beans, but rather to your weakened digestive system. Take Beano® or a generic version of alpha-galactosidase temporarily until your digestive system is stronger.

Fish and seafood can be eaten by people who do not want to be vegetarians. If you look in your mouth you will see we have canine teeth. Humans can eat about one tenth animal food and the best choice is seafood. A few people are allergic to fish and seafood, however, and will not be able to eat them. Just limit seafood to about 10% of your diet. If you want to be a vegetarian or vegan don't eat seafood, as there are no other animal products in the American macrobiotic diet.

We eat twice the protein we need, and this causes many health problems including obesity. Many studies prove a high protein diet raises uric acid, and causes kidney and liver problems. Anytime you hear an author advocating a high protein diet you will know they are ignorant and uninformed. Whole grains, beans and vegetables contain all the high quality protein you need. There are many studies to prove this. At Nara Medical University (Nara Igaku Zasshi v. 46, 1995) the doctors concluded, "A protein-limited diet was useful for prevention of diabetic nephropathy in patients with early-stage diabetic nephropathy." At the University of Vermont (American Journal of Physiology v. 27, 1996) the same results were found; decreased protein intake was found to improve symptoms of type 1 diabetes.

Most all green and yellow vegetables are a good choice if you avoid nightshades, most tropical vegetables, and those high in oxalic acid. Japanese macrobiotics does not include many green and yellow vegetables, ironically. Actually, frozen vegetables are very nutritious; only the texture is harmed by the freezing process. Canned vegetables should be avoided. Avoid the nightshade family which includes potatoes, tomatoes, peppers, and eggplants. Nightshades contain large amounts of toxic solanine. Macrobiotics is about the only diet system to warn against these nightshade vegetables. Also avoid vegetables high in oxalic acid such as spinach, Swiss chard and others. Tropical vegetables like taro, etc. are meant for tropical peoples living in tropical climates. If you are of, say, African or Indian descent living in southern Florida or Arizona you certainly can eat such tropical foods. If you are of European descent these foods were simply not meant for you.

People with blood sugar dysmetabolism cannot eat fruits, fruit juice, dried fruits, or sweeteners of any type until they are well. If your pancreas has atrophied or been removed this means you have to take them out of your diet permanently. You might think fruits provide important nutrients, and your diet will be incomplete without them. This is not the case at all, since fruits are basically made up of simple sugars, fiber and water with very few vitamins and minerals. You cannot use sweeteners including honey, fructose, fruit juice, dried fruit, maple syrup, stevia, lo han, molasses, rice syrup, corn syrup or any others. Sugar is sugar is sugar, and honey is biologically no better than white table sugar. Artificial sweeteners are the worst, and none of them are safe. The newest claim from sucralose to be, "made from sugar, tastes like sugar," is very misleading. They don't tell you this is a manmade halogenated (chlorine molecules are added), synthetic, chemical, unnatural analog that just isn't safe for human use. Kick the sugar habit and take the concept of "desserts" out of your life. You don't need desserts or sweets.

Scientists in Japan concluded, "The main reason of recent increase of diabetic patients is ascribed to increased sucrose intake" (Chiba Igaku Zasshi 72 (1996). Folks, Americans eat more than 160 pounds of various sugars and sweeteners every year which they don't need at all. The worst offender of all is high fructose corn syrup since it is the cheapest to produce. At the Diabetes Research Centre in India (Diabetologica 44, 2001) it was shown the urban (not rural) Indians have an inordinate sugar intake which causes epidemic diabetes rates even though they are largely vegetarian and eat a very low fat diet. Eating sweets will raise your triglyceride levels very much even without eating fats.

It will be difficult for some people to simply give up all sweets and fruits. You can go through a transition period where you eat no cakes, cookies, sodas, pies, candy and the other high sugar foods. For a few months you can eat 10% fresh (not dried or juiced) local fruit. No tropical fruits, as these are meant for tropical peoples in tropical lands- genetics and climate. You can also get a macrobiotic dessert cookbook and make whole grain desserts lightly sweetened with whole fruit only. You'll come to enjoy these and the subtle sweetness will be enough for you. Please remember macrobiotic desserts are a temporary transition, and the sooner you take all fruit and sweeteners out of your diet the faster you'll get well. Your body simply cannot handle simple sugars regardless of how "natural" they are. Honey is still sugar. When you are fully cured you can eat 10% local fresh fruit if you want.

You should enjoy a wide variety of natural soups. Eating soup will help you lose weight and stay slim. That's right, if you eat just two meals a day and start with a delicious bowl of soup at each meal, you'll actually feel full and eat less food. Get some soup cookbooks and learn to substitute healthier ingredients where meat, poultry, eggs and dairy are called for. Traditional Japanese macrobiotics restricted you to only 5% soup daily and almost always miso soup. There is just no reason for these kinds of unnecessary limitations. There is nothing magical or special about fermented soybeans. There are countless delicious soups you can make at home and freeze for future use.

You can eat a fresh, green salad every day as long as you use a low fat, non-dairy dressing. Traditional Japanese macro-biotics had a bias against fresh salads for some reason. In fact they had a bias against any raw foods at all basically. The best time to eat salads is in summer time since they are rather yin. You can still enjoy fresh salads all year round. People who advocate a 100% raw

29

food diet are neurotic and cannot stay on these very long as their health deteriorates so badly.

What about real world, published studies that 1) show the difference it cultural diets and rates of diabetes, and 2) diabetics who are given whole food diets? At Pantox Laboratories in CA (Medical Hypotheses v. 58, 2002) type 2 diabetics were given a natural vegan (no animal products) diet along with daily walking. This study was backed up by a stunning 170 references. "The vegan diet/exercise strategy represents a safe, low-tech approach to managing diabetes that deserves far greater attention from medical researchers and practitioners." The patients got very quick, dramatic improvements and benefits including basic changes in their very blood parameters. They were fed local and tropical fruits which should be omitted. You don't have to be a vegan to do this.

A cross-sectional study was done at the famous Cambridge University (British Journal of Nutrition v. 83, 2000) which concluded, "Healthy Balanced Diets As One of the Main Components of Disease Prevention." 802 people were given GTTs and it was clear the ones who made better food choices had far less diabetes. The healthy people ate more vegetables, salads, fish, fruits, pasta and rice. The ones with poor GTT results ate more sausages, meat, dairy, eggs, and fried foods generally. In another study 25,698 Seventh Day Adventist vegetarians were examined. (American Journal of Public Health v. 75, 1985). Adventists are known to have far less diabetes, cancer, heart disease and other conditions as a whole. The ones who did not eat eggs or dairy products were the healthiest. You can't argue with the results of almost twenty-six thousand real men and women.

Doctors at UCLA gave almost 5,000 male and female diabetics a diet and exercise program (Diabetes Care v. 17, 1994) for just three weeks. Glucose levels fell dramatically. In just 21 days and 71% of the ones taking oral medication discontinued their drugs! *That is over 7 in 10 in 21 days!* 39% of those on insulin stopped injecting themselves! *That is almost 4 in 10 getting off*

30

insulin in 21 days! They simply ate better foods and did some moderate exercise. Imagine what would happen if they did this for a whole year. These results are simply amazing!

We've got to mention the Pima Indians again. Half the Pima Indians still live in Mexico and follow their ancient traditions of diet and lifestyle, while the others live in the southwestern U.S. and have largely adopted the American lifestyle. Many studies have been done here because they are the same genetic stock. This one (Diabetes Care v. 24, 2001) from the University of Pittsburg looked at their diabetes rates. The Mexican Pimas ate more corn, beans, squash, melons and desert plants. They actually ate more calories (they do more physical labor), but had lower glucose levels and far less diabetes. The American Pimas have a 50% diabetes rates, short lifespans and many other diseases from eating the usual high-fat, high sugar, refined food diet. American Pimas given their native diet decrease their disease rates immediately.

A fine review from the Helicon Foundation (Medical Hypotheses v. 54, 2000) with 84 references was titled, "Toward a Wholly Nutritional Therapy for Type 2 Diabetes". The authors suggest preventing and treating type 2 diabetes with only diet, supplements and exercise rather than using toxic, ineffective drugs. They also point out obesity, one of the most important causes of all, would be basically eradicated by such dietary means. We need more such progressive doctors using natural means to cure disease.

Another study from Harvard (Annals of Internal Medicine v. 136, 2002) was titled, "Dietary Patterns and Risk for Type 2 Diabetes in U.S. Men". Here over 42,000 men aged 40-75 were studied for diabetes, cancer and heart disease for twelve years. It was clear the ones who ate more whole grains, vegetables, fresh fruits, and fish lived the longest and had the lowest illness rates. The ones who ate red meat, refined grains, dairy products, fried foods, and desserts had far higher disease rates and much shorter lives. Forty-two thousand real men prove the point conclusively.

The diet books in print are generally terrible, and there are very few authors who have any idea of what they're talking about. If you go to a bookstore or library you will see many books claiming to tell you how to cure diabetes. Nearly all of them are not only useless, but will actually make you worse. You can always tell if the books are spurious if the author suggests eating dairy products, eggs, meat, poultry, sweeteners of any kind (including honey, stevia, etc.), tropical foods (like bananas and citrus), or nightshade vegetables like potatoes and tomatoes. It is not considered "good form" in this business to mention these pseudo-authorities by name, so they won't be named specifically.

Susan Powter has written two good books, *Stop the Insanity* and *Food*, on eating well, staying slim, and calorie density. Susan practices what she preaches and looks great at 47. Neal Barnard is a member of the Physicians Committee for Responsible Medicine (PCRM) and is a very sincere person. His books include *Turn Off the Fat Genes, Live Longer, Live Better, Food for Life, and Eat Right, Live Longer.* Gary Null has written *Get Healthy Now, Vegetarian Handbook,* and *Seven Steps to Perfect Health.* Terry Shintani is a very committed man who wrote *The Hawaii Diet,* and *The Good Carbohydrate Revolution.* Dean Ornish is also a member of the PCRM and has written *Eat More, Weigh Less* and *Program for Reversing Heart Disease.* Robert Pritikin (Nathan Pritikin's son) has written a half dozen books on low fat vegetarian eating. The old Nathan Pritikin books are still available in your public library. Michio Kushi is a prolific writer on traditional Japanese macrobiotics as is George Ohsawa. You should read both of these authors and then take the unnecessary, overly restrictive, limited, obsessive-compulsive Japanese trappings out of their writings. It seems that macrobiotic authors are the only ones to understand such basic truths as the toxicity of nightshade vegetables, and the fact tropical foods aren't meant for temperate peoples. None of the aforementioned authors really understand proven supplements and natural hormone balance to any degree, sorry to say.

The ridiculous "glycemic index" must be mentioned. This

pseudo-scientific silliness is ridiculous on its face. To start with, their standard of reference is white bread! Sadly enough this glycemic absurdity now appears in medical journals! The glycemic theory says that brown rice raises blood sugar as much as a sugared donut, and that a bowl of hearty oatmeal raises blood sugar as much as a Twinkie®. If this was true that whole grains and beans raised blood sugar, the Asian countries would have the highest rates of diabetes in the world! The fact they have the lowest rates proves otherwise. You'll notice that the advocates of the glycemic index suggest eating red meat, poultry, eggs, and dairy products while warning against whole grains and legumes generally. Anyone who promotes the glycemic index is obviously ignorant and should be *ignored.*

Calorie restriction is an important part of curing blood sugar conditions. Americans eat twice the calories they need. We eat three meals a day when we only need two. Be sure to *eat two meals a day* instead of three. You only need to eat twice a day and soon this will become perfectly normal for you. Breakfast is not, "the most important meal of the day." The less you eat the longer you live. We only need two meals a day and no snacks. Men can thrive on about 1,800 calories a day and women on about 1,200 calories. Roy Walford is the only one who wrote extensively on this subject. Please read his *The 120 Year Diet* and *Maximum Lifespan.* Eat as little as possible and keep your caloric intake down by eating low fat foods. It isn't food that makes you fat; *it is fat that makes you fat.* You don't need to walk around hungry, nor can you. Willpower is an illusion. You can eat all you want and still take in very few calories by simply *making better food choices. You can eat all you want and never be hungry and still stay slim if you just eat whole, natural foods.* The answer is in eating lower fat foods and not less food. Please take a good look at the calorie density chart in *Chapter 13: Obesity* to convince yourself you can literally eat all you want if you make better food choices.

It would literally take 80 years to study humans for the total benefits of calorie restriction, but we have 1) shorter term human studies, and 2) full term animal studies. There is no doubt that calorie restriction is the most effective way to extend lifespan and quality of life when a whole foods diet is incorporated. At Heinrich-Heine University in Germany a heavily referenced review was published (Weiner Klinische Wochen v. 106, 1994) where real people greatly improved their insulin sensitivity and lost weight by eating lower calorie foods. At the Franco-Czech Laboratory (Journal of Clinical Endocrinology & Metabolism v. 89, 2002) obese women improved their insulin resistance and lost weight by simply eating lower calorie foods. At Jinan University (Zhongguo Gonggong Weisheng 18, 1994) elderly people ate lower calorie foods and improved their GTT results, lowered their cholesterol and triglycerides with no other changes. At University of California in San Francisco (Diabetes 49, 2000) obese people ate low calorie foods, lost weight, lost body fat, and improved glucose metabolism in only 20 days! Imagine the results for the rest of your life. At Alexandra Hospital (International Journal of Obesity v. 27, 2003) obese diabetic men were given lower calorie foods for 12 weeks. They lost weight, lost body fat, lowered their cholesterol, and improved glycemic control very much with no other intervention. At Nagasaki University (International Congress Series v.1209, 2000) diabetic women were fed a low calorie, low fat diet based on rice and vegetables. Their glycemic status improved and their glucose levels fell significantly.

Fasting is always a part of any serious natural health program. Unfortunately, with most blood sugar disorders you cannot do well for a day or more on water without any food. Therefore we will not discuss fasting or recommend the many good books on the values and benefits. The books on fasting are listed in *Zen Macrobiotics for Americans.* When you are cured it is important you fast one day a week on water from dinner to dinner. This gives your body 52 times every year to rest, recuperate and heal. Once you see the great benefits you'll probably choose to do longer fasts. It is unfortunate that people with blood sugar problems generally can't even fast for 24 hours without discomfort.

Chapter 6: Effective Supplements

It cannot be repeated enough that *what you eat* is the real cure for blood sugar and insulin dysmetabolism. Your daily food is what will cure you basically. Whole natural foods cure disease. Proven supplements and natural hormones are powerful, but only secondary to diet. People are understandably confused about which supplements work and which are merely advertising promotions. This confusion can be explained in one word - *advertising*. To know which supplements honestly have value we merely need to look at *the scientific literature* rather than the very well written advertisements that inundate us. *Science* tells us which supplements really benefit us, not skillful ad writers.

First, we need to understand the difference between "endogenous" supplements and "exogenous" ones. Endogenous supplements exist in our bodies and in the common foods we eat. This would include all vitamins, all minerals, all basic hormones, most amino acids, and such supplements as CoQ10, beta sitosterol, lipoic acid, DIM, PS, and beta glucan. You can and should take the appropriate and needed endogenous supplements the rest of your life for your general health, especially if you are over forty. Exogenous supplements do not exist naturally in our bodies nor in our common foods. This would include such things as herbs in general (e.g. ginseng, echinacea, milk thistle, golden seal, etc.), green tea, curcumin, guggul, ellagic acid and aloe vera. Even if any of these supplements are appropriate for you, the effect will only last for about six months to a year and then cease. To continue taking them would be a waste of time and money and could even be counterproductive. Many people are, in fact, allergic to some of these exogenous products. Therefore, we will stress long term endogenous supplements, but still mention the temporary exogenous ones for short term use.

Lipoic acid has so much research on it there is a separate chapter *(Chapter 8: Lipoic Acid)* devoted to the many international published studies on its benefits.

You should take any good, reliable brand of multivitamins. There are only thirteen vitamins and all have an established RDA (recommended daily allowance). Never take megadoses of any vitamin (or other supplement) as these overdoses unbalance our metabolism. Regular *vitamin B-12* is absorbed very poorly, so pick a supplement with 1 mg of methylcobalamin as the preferred form of B-12. Minerals are so important they are covered in separate chapter (*Chapter 9: The Minerals We Need*).

Vitamin C is a very overrated and misunderstood vitamin, and megadoses of this will acidify your normally alkaline blood. Making the blood pH acidic causes your entire system to be sickly. Megadoses of *anything* - including oxygen, sun, fun, food, sex, or whatever else - are harmful. You should understand that vitamin C is only basically found in any quantity in tropical fruits, such as citrus, which are meant for tropical people in hot climates. You find very little vitamin C in temperate climate fruits and vegetables. Diabetics use up excessive vitamin C due to the increased need for all antioxidants. Therefore you should take 250 mg until you are well. You can continue to take 250 mg after you are well if you want as the RDA is 60 mg. Studies at Myong Ji University in Korea, Showa University in Japan, Harvard Medical School, Semmelweis University in Hungary, Zagazig University in Egypt, and the CDC in Atlanta have all shown increased need for vitamin C in diabetes. Again, do not take more than 250 mg, as this is four times the RDA- Linus Pauling was wrong! Short term studies of megadoses of vitamin C may show limited benefits, but never in the long term.

Beta glucan is a very important supplement to take for all forms of sugar dysmetabolism. The usual dosage is 200 mg, but you should take 400 mg for the first year to improve glycemic control. Beta glucan is *the* most powerful immune enhancer known to science including interferon-alpha. It doesn't matter whether you use oat or yeast glucan as all are 1/3 true glucans. The mushroom glucan is simply too expensive. Please read my book *What Is Beta Glucan?* to learn more. A good number of animal studies showed the benefits of beta glucan for diabetes, and finally human studies were done to verify these. At the Centre for Food and Animal Research in Canada (Carbohydrate Polymers v. 25, 1994) humans were given oat beta glucan to help normalize their blood sugar and insulin levels. At the University of Vienna in Austria (Journal of Pediatric Gastroenterotology v.32, 2001) diabetic children were given beta glucan to improve their blood sugar metabolism. At the University of Lausanne in Switzerland (European Journal of Clinical Nutrition 55, 2001) healthy men were given beta glucan, which greatly improved their glucose and insulin levels. Beta glucan also has powerful cholesterol and triglyceride lowering activity which, of course, is of great concern in blood sugar dysmetabolism. This is a very important supplement you must add to your regimen and even healthy children and young people should routinely take this.

Ironically the carotenoid *beta carotene* has been shown to be deficient in most diabetics, but not vitamin A. (Beta carotene is the direct precursor to vitamin A.) Beta carotene is one of the most powerful antioxidants in our diet. In fact, some studies, such as the one done at Jikei University in Japan, show high serum vitamin A levels, but low levels of beta carotene. You only need 10,000 IU here, although you can take 25,000 for the first year if you want to. This is a very effective antioxidant and should definitely be a part of your program. The Third National Health and Nutrition Examination Survey (Diabetes v. 52, 2003) showed low levels of carotenoids (except lycopene, of course, which is a promotional fraud) generally in diabetics.

CoQ10 is a basic supplement here and you must take 100 mg a day. Some unscrupulous companies offer smaller amounts with "special delivery systems" that are all but worthless. 100 mg is what you need. Some "experts" recommend 300 to 400 mg a day, but this is a waste of money and not necessary at all. Real Japanese bioengineered CoQ10 is about $4,000 per kilogram in

2005. You can find bottles of 60 X 100 mg for under $40. Do not use cheaper, inferior products made from tobacco plants such as the ones sold in membership clubs for under $20. At Royal Perth Hospital in Australia (European Journal of Clinical Nutrition v. 56, 2002), it was concluded, "CoQ10 supplementation may improve blood pressure and long-term glycemic control in subjects with type 2 diabetes." At the same hospital (Diabetologica v.45, 2002) type 2 diabetic patients were much improved with CoQ10 supplementation especially hypertension, glycemic control, and endothelial function. A third study at Perth (Atherosclerosis v.168, 2003) found similar improvements in patients. Diabetics at Odense University in Denmark (Molecular Aspects of Medicine v.18, 1997) found glucose lowering effects of CoQ10 in type 1 diabetics. At Moradabad Hospital in India (Antioxidants in Human Health and Disease 1999) a review with 59 references on the benefits of CoQ10 for diabetes and CHD was published.

At the NKP Salve Institute in India (Journal of Human Hypertension 13, 1999) patients on various medications were given 120 mg of CoQ10 daily for 8 weeks. Their blood pressure fell significantly. Their insulin levels fell from 465 pmol to 257! Their glucose fell from 7.86 mmol to 5.26. Their triglycerides also fell considerably. Remember this was with no change in diet or other factors. A heavily referenced review (Medical Hypotheses v.52, 1999) also demonstrated the value of CoQ10 for diabetes, especially for improving beta cell function.

Beta-sitosterol is found in every vegetable you eat, but there just isn't enough in our daily food. It is estimated the average American eats about 300 mg daily, while vegetarians eat twice that amount. Vegetarians have far less blood sugar problems. Take 300 mg a day of mixed sterols (mixed sterols is the only form available). You should take 600 mg a day for the first year and then just 300 mg. Beta-sitosterol is the most effective natural remedy known for both prostate problems and high blood fats (cholesterol and triglycerides). At the Gerontology Clinic (Vnitrni Lekarstvi v. 50, 2004) blood levels of these plant sterols were shown to be very important in diabetic patients. "In diabetics the level of disease compensation correlated negatively with plant sterol values." Similar studies were done at the University of Stellenbosch in South Africa (Current Opinion in Clinical Nutrition v. 4, 2001). Obese people and type 2 diabetics were shown to have low serum plant sterol levels at the University of Helsinki in Finland (Obesity Research v. 10, 2002). All this is strongly related to cholesterol and triglyceride dysmetabolism.

Acetyl-L-carnitine (ALC) is the preferred form of L-carnitine as it is more bioavailable, and passes into the brain more easily. 500 mg a day is the appropriate dose. There are a number of studies on both forms, but you will get all the benefits of plain L-carnitine by taking the acetyl derivative ALC. At the Instituto di Medicina in Italy (Metabolism v. 49, 2000) type 2 diabetics were given ALC which effectively increased their glucose disposal and utilization. They concluded this was an important therapy. Numerous animal studies have been done with ALC showing good benefits. More studies have been done on L-carnitine itself on both animals and humans. ALC is an important supplement for anyone over 40 for brain function, memory and clarity of thought.

Vitamin D is not a vitamin at all, but rather a hormone. It does not occur in our food except small amounts in a few animal foods such as eggs. This is *the* most important "vitamin" of all for blood sugar problems. Your daily vitamin supplement should have 400 IU, but you should take another 400 IU for many reasons. You should be getting a total of 800 IU of vitamin D unless you are out in the sun a lot. In the summer, if you get regular exposure to the sun, you can just take the 400 IU in your vitamin supplement. Most Americans are clearly deficient in "vitamin" D generally as most of us do not get out in the sun regularly, especially in winter months. Science proves that low serum vitamin D levels are critical in many illnesses, especially many forms of cancer. The international research on vitamin D and blood sugar is very strong.

The best review of vitamin D and Syndrome X was done at

Royal London Hospital (British Journal of Nutrition v. 79, 1998) with 13 pages and over 140 references. "Evidence is presented suggesting that vitamin D deficiency may be an avoidable risk factor for Syndrome X." At Boston University (American Journal of Clinical Nutrition v. 79, 2003) a review was published showing vitamin D supplementation helps prevent common cancers, diabetes, heart disease and osteoporosis. There are numerous other reviews and studies to support this.

Vitamin E is the second most important vitamin for blood sugar problems. Vitamin E is also very deficient in our diets because whole grains - the main source - are so rarely eaten. Always use the *natural mixed* tocopherols and not the inexpensive single tocopherol (d-alpha). Be sure to use the mixed natural form for a few dollars more. You can even use 200 IU a day effectively, or up to 400 IU daily. Do not exceed this since the RDA is only 30 IU. The research on this is simply overwhelming and cannot possibly be covered. Vitamin E is one of the most powerful of all natural antioxidants and must be a part of your healing program.

Hunan Medical University gave vitamin E to type 2 diabetics with dramatic benefits in only 30 days. The University of Chieti in Italy showed significant benefits in only 14 days in type 2 diabetics. The same thing happened at the University of Texas in 90 days. The Postgraduate Institute in India got better glycemic control in only 4 weeks. Type 1 diabetics at University Clinic Ulm in Germany responded well after 6 months. Type 1 diabetics improved in 90 days at Monash Medical Center in Australia. A mere 100 IU of vitamin E improved type 1 diabetics and lowered their triglycerides in only 90 days. The Louisiana State University doctors found the same benefits with only 100 IU. The University of Naples in Italy did a review of the literature and concluded vitamin E supplementation should be standard practice. The research here is obviously overwhelming and we couldn't possibly quote it all. In 2005 the medical profession tried to discredit the value of vitamin E supplementation with spurious "studies".

Flaxseed oil is the best source of omega-3 fatty acids, and better than fish oil for a lot of reasons. All the studies on fish oil apply equally to flax oil since the omega-3 content is basically the same. Regardless of your age, be sure to take at least 1,000 mg a day of flax oil. Even if you eat fish regularly you'll never get the amounts you need. Buy and keep this refrigerated - do not buy unrefrigerated flax oil as it easily oxidizes. We eat far too much omega-6 fatty acids and far too few omega-3s, so take 1-2 grams a day. The research is overwhelming on the benefits of omega-3 supplementation especially for heart and artery health and blood lipids. The benefits here are not for insulin and glucose metabolism per se, but more for blood lipids especially triglycerides.

At Federico II University in Italy type 2 diabetics were given omega-3 supplements which lowered their triglycerides and improved their blood parameters. At the same University diabetics will hypertriglyceridemia lowered their levels from 3.85 mmol to only 2.92 in 60 days using no other therapies. At the National Institute of Public Health in Norway women who took omega-3 supplements had children with far less genetic diabetes. At Barzilai Medical Center in Israel hypertensive, obese and dyslipidemic people with and without diabetes were given omega-3 supplements with impressive results. The Center for Genetics in Washington, DC did a review with a full 98 references on essential fatty acids. This showed we eat excessive omega-6 and deficient omega-3 fatty acids which are a major cause of heart and artery disease, diabetes, cancer and other illnesses. At the Univesity of Milano in Italy patients lowered their triglycerides in only 60 days by simply taking an omega-3 supplement with no other treatment. The Sri Venkateswara University in India concluded that supplementation with omega-3 fatty acids had beneficial effects on serum triglycerides, HDL cholesterol, lipid peroxidation and antioxidant enzymes, which can lead to decreased rate of occurrence of vascular complications of diabetes. The Center for Diabetes in Italy found omega-3 administration appeared advisable in insulin dependant diabetics with increased CHD risk factors. The research here is too much to continue with. Take at least one gram of flax oil daily regardless of your age.

L-glutamine is a proven amino acid for good intestinal health. You should take a gram (two X 500 mg) in the AM and another gram in the PM. This will also spike (but not raise for a whole day) your growth hormone levels. While L-glutamine has shown no specific value for blood sugar problems, always remember we are treating *the whole body* and not just our glucose metabolism. Regardless of our age, our digestive systems are generally in terrible shape from our poor diets. Taking L-glutamine with a good brand of acidophilus and FOS will help us digest our food well. Strong digestion is an important part of maintaining normal blood sugar and insulin levels.

FOS is fructooligosaccarides. This is an indigestible sugar that feeds the good bacteria in our intestines, but not the "bad" bacteria. This will not help blood sugar dysmetabolism directly, but will help keep your intestines healthy to better digest your food which helps normalize glucose metabolism. Taking 750 mg once or twice a day works very well with acidophilus and L-glutamine to keep our digestive system strong and healthy.

Acidophilus keeps the good bacteria in our intestines alive. Find a good refrigerated brand and keep it refrigerated. Take 3 billion units once or twice daily and use FOS and L-glutamine with it. This will help you digest your food better.

PS is phosphatidyl serine and a relative of lecithin or phosphatidyl choline. Only in the last few years has inexpensive PS become available to the public, and the human research verified its value. Take 100 mg a day if you are over the age of 40 to support good brain function. This is not going to help glycemic control per se, but you are treating your total health and not just glucose metabolism. Pregnenolone and acetyl-L-carnitine work very well with PS. You can also benefit from taking a 1,200 mg softgel of lecithin for both better brain metabolism and lower cholesterol and triglyceride levels.

Glucosamine will not specifically help your blood sugar condition, but it is an important supplement for anyone over the age of 40. Literally 95% of Americans over the age of 65 suffer from arthritis and joint inflammation. Glucosamine 500 mg a day is a proven supplement for bone and joint health. Do not take chondroitin as it is not absorbed by our intestines and is therefore useless. Glucosamine cannot work alone and must have a complete supply of minerals, flax oil and vitamin D to be effective.

Superoxide dismutase (SOD) is one of our two main antioxidant enzymes. Unfortunately we cannot take oral SOD pills, nasal sprays are illegal, sublingual SOD isn't available, nor is the use of DMSO transdermal solutions. Doctors don't know how to inject this, and it wouldn't be practical anyway. Nevertheless, SOD is very important to blood sugar problems because of the antioxidant stress. The University of Tiemcen in Algeria found low SOD blood levels in type 2 (but not in type 1) diabetics. Hyogo University in Japan found low SOD in type 1.

What can we do? Fortunately we can keep our SOD levels elevated with diet, supplements, lifestyle, and generally supporting our antioxidant defense system. By taking all the supplements listed in this chapter you will be supporting the natural production of SOD. By eating well, exercising, balancing your basic hormones and avoiding negative habits (such as coffee, alcohol, cigarettes, recreational drugs) you will have a higher level of SOD. If the nasal, sublingual, or transdermal in DMSO forms of SOD were legalized we could simply take them. SOD creams and sprays are available, but these are not transdermal and will not go into your bloodstream. Any oral SOD product should be avoided despite the claims of "special delivery systems", etc.

Glutathione is our other basic antioxidant enzyme. You can take oral glutathione, but it is not as effective as NAC. NAC is *N-acetyl cysteine* and is a much more effective way to raise your glutathione levels than glutathione itself. Take 600 mg a day. You can choose to continue this or stop taking it after you are cured.

The conventional wisdom that glutathione blood levels fall dramatically as we age just isn't correct, and they only fall about 10% in most people. In diabetic conditions, however, glutathione has been shown to be of great importance due to it being so basic to our antioxidant process. This is a vital supplement for blood sugar conditions and much research has been done here.

Soy isoflavones can be taken in 40 mg doses of combined genestein and diadzein. It is naïve to think we are going to get a sufficient intake of these valuable isoflavones by eating a variety of soy products. An eight ounce glass of soy milk daily will supply what you need, but will also add about 120 calories to your daily intake. Tofu is the white bread of soybeans, is highly refined, and lacking in nutrition. Westerners rarely eat any amount of soy products such as miso, seitan, soy flour, tempeh or other traditional Asian foods. Soy sauce is merely a condiment. There is an overwhelming amount of published research on the benefits of soy supplementation. Anyone who tells you soy is "bad" for you is mentally deficient. The dairy and meat industries are very upset by the popularity of soy products especially soy milks.

DIM (di-indolylmethane) is a fine supplement which is stronger and cheaper than I3C (indole-3-carbinol) for lowering and improving estrogen metabolism. Take 200 mg of DIM daily. If you test your free estradiol and estrone levels and find them to be in the normal range you won't need to take this. Men over the age of 50 generally have higher estradiol and estrone levels than their postmenopausal wives! Excess estrogen in men or women is harmful and upsets the actions of the other hormones including insulin. American and European women rarely have insufficient estrogen levels due to their high fat, low fiber, nutrient deficient diets, obesity and lack of exercise among other factors. Asian women who have lower estradiol and estrone (but not estriol) levels have less heart disease, osteoporosis and menopausal problems. The idea that American women generally are somehow "estrogen deficient" after menopause is simply not true.

Chapter 7: Temporary Supplements

There are a variety of temporary supplements to take for up to a year. Most of these are "exogenous" and not in our bodies or in our common food. The rest are endogenous (in our bodies and common food), but just not needed after about a year.

TMG (betaine) or trimethylglycine is the most powerful liver rejuvenator known. Taking 3 grams a day (6 X 500 mg capsules) for a year will do wonders to cleanse and strengthen your liver. Liver problems, especially such conditions as fatty liver, are usually central to blood sugar problems. While TMG is endogenous, there is just no reason to use this for more than a year. This is a very important temporary supplement you should add to your healing program. The human studies are excellent.

Vitamin C was covered in the previous chapter. It must be emphasized that megadoses weaken your immunity in the long run. It is *not* a dietary deficiency of vitamin C here at all, but rather the fact the body is using up all the vitamin C and other antioxidants it can get to balance the free radicals. You should only take 250 mg or less a day and *never* take megadoses. Therefore large doses of vitamin C are *not* going to be a temporary supplement for you.

Aloe vera is a classic healing herb that helps our digestive system and our liver among other benefits. Taking 2 X 100 mg capsules of a 200:1 extract is easier than trying to drink the equivalent of 40 grams of fresh gel. Aloe gel is 99.5% water.

Ellagic acid has no proof of efficacy for blood sugar disorders per se, but has shown very powerful anti-cancer and other effects. Taking 100 mg a day for one year will help your immunity in general.

Milk thistle is the most effective herb for liver health. Taking 2 capsules of a good extract every day for one year will work with the TMG to strengthen your liver. Milk thistle is the most researched herb for liver health, but is exogenous and will not help you after using it for about a year or less. There are many human studies on the active ingredient silymarin.

Taurine has a lot of science behind it finally for humans and diabetes. Numerous animal studies showed great promise here, and now the human studies verify this. Take 500 mg of taurine daily for one year. This inexpensive amino acid also has much value for coronary heart conditions generally and helps lower blood fats and blood pressure. Beijing Hospital in China, Cardiology Research Center in Moscow, Bengbu Medical College in China, and Research University in Italy all showed improvement in glucose levels, insulin sensitivity, blood parameters, and other benefits in both type 1 and 2 diabetes. Studies at the University of Messina, and the Diabetes Unit in Italy, showed diabetics had low blood plasma and platelet taurine levels. In 2004 an extensive review of the literature with 114 references from the University of Sassari in Italy showed that taurine supplementation is valuable in treating diabetes and insulin resistance.

Curcumin taken in 500 mg amounts daily for one year is a powerful and proven natural antioxidant.

Green tea extract is very worthwhile. Just take two capsules daily. Green tea is simply regular old tea (Thea sinensis) that is not fermented. There is a lot of good research on green tea polyphenols, but all of it is short term only. This is an exogenous food, and the fact it *must* have the caffeine removed to be safe is rather worrisome. It is unlikely you will drink two cups of de-caf green tea every day, so the capsules are much more practical.

Quercitin is technically an endogenous antioxidant although basically only found in apples and onions. You can take 100 mg daily for one year. Only one study was found where diabetic rats much improved by quercitin supplementation.

Polysaccharide plant gums such as *glucomannon*, *guar gum*, *pectin* (citrus or apple), and *sodium alginate* (from seaweed) are very valuable, inexpensive, and safe temporary supplements. These gums have shown value in lowering cholesterol, blood sugar normalization, and other benefits. Take at least 3 grams a day (6 X 500 mg capsules) to get real benefit. Choose the one you prefer, the one that is least expensive, or try each of the four above for three month periods successively. The added rewards of lowering cholesterol and triglycerides will be an important factor in your healing as well. Some people have lost weight using these since these gums swell up dramatically with water and fill the stomach giving you a feeling of having eaten when you haven't. The science here is very strong. "Modified" citrus pectin is a fraud.

At the 7th annual Gums and Stabilizers Conference in England researchers reviewed the benefits of these and found, "improved glycemic control and a reduction in plasma cholesterol," which, of course, are precursors to diabetes. At the University of Helsinki a review with 59 references was published showing guar gum therapy had favorable long-term effects on glycemic control and lipid levels in NIDDM subjects. At St. Marianna University in Japan (Eiyogaku Zasshi v. 56, 1998) galactomannon (from fenugreek) was found to benefit by feeding five grams a day to type 2 diabetics. At the Institute of Investigations in Cuba guar, pectin and glucomannon were all shown to help remove toxic heavy metals from the blood, improve digestion generally and lessen the effects of diabetes.

L-arginine is an overrated and promoted amino acid with little scientific evidence behind it. There are a few studies, however, for blood sugar conditions. You can use 3 grams (6 X 500 mg) daily for one year. At the University of Vienna L-arginine was found to inhibit lipid peroxidation in human diabetics. At the Medical College of Wisconsin diabetic rats benefited from L-arginine in their water. At Cumhuriyet University in Turkey rabbits lowered blood glucose levels with oral L-arginine.

Asian or American *ginseng* can be used temporarily, but not in hot weather or in tropical climates because of its extreme yang (warm) nature. Find a reliable brand and take one or two capsules a day during the coolest six months of the year (October thru March in the Northern Hemisphere).

Nopal cactus has been promoted for normalizing blood sugar levels, but where is the evidence? There are no human or animal studies published in any of the international medical journals. There is just no reason to use something unproven like this when you have so many proven supplements to use. Bitter melon (Momordica) has also been promoted for blood sugar problems, but again where is the evidence? Banaba leaf has corosolic acid in it and has been promoted for blood sugar problems. The published evidence is just not convincing so far. Fenugreek herb (containing galactomannon fiber) has been commercially promoted for diabetes, but the science is lacking here, too. Conjugated linoleic acid (CLA) has been promoted for weight loss as well as diabetes, but, again, the evidence isn't there.

The herb most promoted for normalizing blood sugar is *Gymnema sylvestre*. There are a good number of animal studies which do show a lot of potential, but almost no human studies at all. There is no reason more human research hasn't been done. Animal studies can be very valuable, and we may see human research done in the next few years. You can certainly use this for a year if you want, but remember that exogenous supplements will not work for some people and will be biologically incompatible (allergenic) in others. If you feel any of these temporary supplements are not compatible with your individual biochemistry then drop them. Some people will get mild side effects from exogenous supplements like these instead of benefits.

Chapter 8: Alpha Lipoic Acid

Lipoic acid (aka thioctic acid) is a natural antioxidant in our bodies, and the most important single supplement you can take for diabetes and blood sugar disorders. There are very small amounts of lipoic acid in our daily food in the form of lipoyllysine, and it does not exist in the free form in our bodies. Do not think this is somehow a Magic Supplement that can work alone. Diet and exercise is the basic cure for blood sugar dysmetabolism, while supplements and hormones play a secondary role. The research on lipoic acid is rather overwhelming, so we are going to devote a separate chapter to it.

Actually lipoic acid is a disulfide (two sulfur atoms) that is converted in the body to dihydro lipoic acid or DHLA. The lipoic acid of commerce and the one used in nearly all the studies is equally composed of two mirror image isomers R- and S-. Most all of the published studies use the regular natural R/S form. You will see Internet advertisements claiming that only the R-isomer has biological value, while the S-isomer is somehow ineffective. Of course, the R- only product is very expensive. Since the regular, normal form sold is 50% R- isomer you would save money by simply using twice as much if you want to believe these pseudo-scientific claims. Please do not be taken in by such unscientific promotions. Clinical studies using these R- and S- forms separately found that they equally convert to DHLA in the body.

Anyone over the age of forty should take lipoic acid as part of their basic supplement program for its powerful antioxidant properties. For most people taking 200 mg a day is sufficient. Clinical studies have used up to 1,000 mg, but only in the short term. Injected lipoic acid is much more effective than oral use, but very impractical obviously. Overdoses of lipoic acid or anything else merely unbalance our metabolism and are contraindicated. If you have a serious problem you can safely take 400 mg a day for one year by using 200 mg in the AM and another 200 mg in the

49

PM to maintain maximum blood levels. Lipoic acid is safe, inexpensive, and non-toxic, but there just isn't any reason to take more than this for the long term. Short term studies have used higher doses, but you'll be doing long term therapy.

At Eberhard-Karls University in Germany (BioFactors 10, 1993) a study, Thioctic Acid-Effects on Insulin Sensitivity and Glucose-Metabolism" was done. They pointed out that, "Thioctic acid is a co-factor of key mitochondrial enzymes, involved in the regulation of glucose oxidation, such as the pyruvate dehydrogenase and the alpha-ketoglutarate dehydrogenase, both enzyme complexes which are known to be diminished in diabetes." In plain words, this means lipoic acid works with our bodies enzymes to prevent glucose from being oxidized. Their conclusion was, "The clinical and experimental date indicate that this compound has beneficial effects on insulin sensitivity, correcting several metabolic pathways known to be altered in type 2 diabetes, such as insulin stimulated glucose uptake, glucose oxidation, and glycogen synthesis." The authors quote two human studies published in Diabetologica 1995 and Arzneimittelforschung 1995. *Here insulin sensitivity was increased 27 to 51% in merely 10 days!* This is nothing less than incredible! No toxic prescription drugs can even start to approach results like that.

At the University of Southern California (Nutrition 17, 2001) "Molecular Aspects of Lipoic Acid in the Prevention of Diabetes Complications" was published. People with diabetes suffer from an endless list of complications eventually ending in premature death. These include vascular (heart and artery) disease, cataracts, retinopathy (vision loss), neuropathy (nerve deterioration) and nephropathy (loss of kidney function). "Available data strongly suggest that LA, because of its antioxidant properties, is particularly suited to the prevention and/or treatment of diabetic complications..... In addition to its antioxidant properties, LA increases glucose uptake.....Further, recent trials have demonstrated that LA improves glucose disposal in patients with type 2 diabetes. In experimental and clinical studies, LA markedly reduced the symptoms of diabetic pathologies, including cataract formation, vascular damage and polyneuropathy." Rather powerful statements.

A most impressive seventeen page, heavily documented review, "The Pharmacology of the Antioxidant Lipoic Acid", from Vrije University in Amsterdam (General Pharmacology v. 29, 1997) leaves no doubt about its effectiveness. Here they prove that the R- and S- isomers equally convert to DHLA in humans. This review is about the antioxidant properties of LA for general health rather than the benefits for diabetes specifically. The language here is highly technical and refers to reactive oxygen species (ROS), NADH, chelation, oxidative stress, and other such topics. In plain English, they show LA supplements to be a most powerful and proven antioxidant that has many benefits as we age.

At the University of Maastricht in the Netherlands (Oxidative Stress and Disease v. 6, 2001) an excellent review was done on the antioxidant properties and therapeutic potential of lipoic acid. "LA can be used in the treatment of type 2 diabetes mellitus and has been shown to increase cellular glucose uptake and utilization." They point out that both the reduced (DHLA) and oxidized (LA) forms have powerful antioxidant properties.

At the University of Arizona (Oxidative Stress and Disease v. 8, 2002) a long, well documented review was done on hyperglycemia and insulin resistance. They strongly suggest using LA as a therapy for both conditions. Further they discuss the underlying mechanisms for using LA in diabetic and pre-diabetic conditions so we can better understand how it is so effective. At Oregon State University (Current Medicinal Chemistry v. 11, 2004) a review was done showing the power of LA to help ameliorate the pathophysiologies of many chronic diseases, and not just diabetes and other forms of blood sugar dysmetabolism.

Diabetic neuropathy (aka polyneuropathy) is caused by the peroxidation of nervous tissues. Many studies show this can be strongly mitigated by lipoic acid supplements alone. For example, at the Diabetes Center in Romania lipoic acid was given to diabetics for 70 days. They found antioxidant therapy with LA improved and may prevent diabetic neuropathy. This improvement was associated with a reduction in indexes of lipid peroxidation. Again in Romania young type 1 diabetics (mean age of 38) were given lipoic acid for 60 days. Their results demonstrated that LA appeared to be an effective drug in the treatment of different forms of autonomic diabetic neuropathy. There was also a dramatic decrease in systolic blood pressure with no other treatment than the LA. At Goethe University in Germany both type 1 and type 2 diabetics were given lipoic acid for only 3 weeks. Their results demonstrated that therapy with LA had a positive influence on the impaired neurovascular reflex arc in patients with diabetic neuropathy.

At the Diabetic Research Institute in Germany an extensive review with 38 references was done on treating people with diabetic polyneuropathy and cardiac autonomic neuropathy with lipoic acid. At Heine University in Germany diabetics were given lipoic acid for only 3 weeks. Their NIS scores improved greatly. The results of their meta-analysis provided evidence that treatment with lipoic acid over 3 weeks was safe and significantly improved both positive neuropathic symptoms and neuropathic deficits to a clinically meaningful degree in diabetic patients with symptomatic polyneuropathy. Also at Heine an extensive, heavily referenced 17 page review was published. Here they showed that lipoic acid is the single most effective supplement for treating oxidative stress in diabetics. At the Royal Pharmacy in England another good review was done. Lipoic acid is now used in Germany for the treatment of diabetic naturopathy and definitive evidence of efficacy should arise from surveillance studies. Lipoic acid may be more effective as a long-term dietary supplement aimed at the prophylactic protection of diabetics from complications.

The Medical Research Institute in California published a study on oxidative stress in type 2 diabetes and lipoic acid. Studies with antioxidants such as vitamin E, lipoic acid, and N-acetyl cysteine are new strategies now available to treat such conditions. At the University of Medicine in Italy diabetics with "burning mouth syndrome" were successfully treated with lipoic acid. Burning mouth syndrome is one common form of neuropathy. Improvement was found in only 60 days and was maintained in over 70% of the patients after one year.

At the University of Heidelberg in Germany diabetic patients were given lipoic acid for 3 months. This data provided evidence that treatment with LA improves significantly the imbalance between increased oxidative stress and depleted antioxidant defense even in patients with poor glycemic control and albuminuria. Later at the same university both type 1 and 2 diabetics we given long term lipoic acid for eighteen months. The results were very good as always with thrombomodulin and urinary albumin concentrations falling impressively with no other treatments. Both of these are important markers for diagnosis of diabetic states. At Oregon State University a 12 page review with extensive references found that lipoic acid therapy was helpful not only for diabetes, but also other diseases associated with oxidative stress. LA was found to be an effective agent to ameliorate certain pathophysiologies of many chronic diseases. A similar review was also done at Oregon State where the evidence was examined for the effectiveness of lipoic acid against such diverse age-related disorders as unwarranted apoptosis (programmed cell death), cardiovascular disease, and cataract formation. The famous Mayo Clinic in Minnesota did a most impressive 16 page review complete with 77 references on lipoic acid that leaves no doubt as to the proven effectiveness on any disease associated with oxidative stress including blood sugar disorders generally. At the University of California in Berkeley another good review with 34 references was done on the properties of lipoic acid in relation to oxidative stress and disease.

At the University of California in Los Angeles a sophist-icated review with an impressive 78 citations was done on the general antioxidant and pro-oxidant properties of lipoic acid. They showed both lipoic acid and dihydrolipoic acid exhibit direct free radical scavenging properties. Other studies provide evidence that lipoic acid supplementation has pro-oxidant properties, decreases oxidative stress, and restores reduced levels of other antioxidants in real people.

At City Hospital in Germany type 1 diabetics were given lipoic acid in order to improve insulin sensitivity. They found oral administration of LA resulted in a significant increase of insulin-stimulated glucose disposal in NIDDM. Better glucose disposal is a clear marker of improvement in blood sugar dysmetabolism. An article in a 1998 issue of Alternative Medicine review found lipoic acid has the potential to prevent diabetes, influence glucose control, and prevent chronic hyperglycemia associated with complications such as neuropathy and cataracts. At Aston University in England diabetics were given vitamin E, vitamin C and lipoic acid. After only six weeks they found the total antioxidant status (TAS) measurement indicated that diabetic blood plasma antioxidant capacity was improved from mere dietary antioxidant supplementation. When you take a variety of proven antioxidants like this they all work synergistically in concert together and the total effectiveness is greatly increased.

There are many other published human studies from around the world on the benefits of oral lipoic acid supplementation for blood sugar and insulin metabolism. Make this a part of your supplement program.

Chapter 9: We All Need Minerals

We're all mineral deficient, every one of us. No matter how well you eat or what supplements you take, you're still lacking in some of the vital elements you need. Our soils are depleted of minerals. Our food lacks minerals. We don't eat well anyway. Please read my book *The Minerals You Need* to learn about the essential minerals that science has shown us we need in our bodies but don't get. This is the most researched and comprehensive book ever written on minerals and is very easy to read. There are 96 natural elements, but modern medicine only recognizes ten of them as essential. This is irrational and defies logic. While sodium, potassium, phosphorous and sulfur are all essential elements, we get enough of these in our food. Let's look at the minerals we are known to need more of.

Calcium is very misunderstood. The idea that we need 1,000 mg a day is ridiculous, and the official government RDA is not based on science whatsoever. The only abundant source of calcium is dairy products, and at least two thirds of the world's population does not include dairy foods in their diet. You cannot possibly get 1,000 mg of calcium a day without eating dairy foods. You should not eat dairy foods because of the lactose (milk sugar) content. All adults of all races are lactose intolerant - period. Americans and Europeans eat more calcium than anyone on earth, yet have the highest rates of bone and joint disease especially arthritis and osteoporosis. Obviously calcium intake isn't the problem, but rather calcium *absorption*. You need at the minimum magnesium, boron, silicon, strontium and vitamin D in order to *absorb* the calcium, and aren't getting enough of these nutrients. There are certainly other nutritional factors in calcium absorption we haven't discovered yet. Taking 250 mg a day of any common, inexpensive calcium salts such as citrates and carbonates is sufficient. Overdosing yourself on calcium is irresponsible and won't benefit you - more is not better.

Magnesium is *the* most studied and most important element in diabetes, and there is overwhelming research behind it. Magnesium is vitally important for our total health since we're generally deficient in it. One in seven Americans is seriously deficient according to blood analysis studies. The major source of magnesium is whole grains, yet almost all of the grain we eat is refined. The RDA is 400 mg, so taking 200 mg or more of any common salts such as citrates, lactates or oxides is sufficient. There is much evidence that magnesium is critical to blood sugar and insulin metabolism as well as outright diabetes.

Iron is very important as it is the "heme" in blood hemoglobin. Women need more than men, and studies consistently show that Americans are generally iron deficient especially women, vegetarians and the elderly. People with diabetes often have a problem excreting iron and end up with excessive blood levels of it. This does not mean you have to take an iron free supplement, but you should be careful not to take more than 18 mg a day. Since you won't be eating red meat and animal products your intake of iron will fall dramatically. The media misreported (as usual) this situation and claimed excess dietary iron was somehow a common problem. This is a rare condition which is not due to excessive intake, but rather inability to get rid of unneeded iron. Men need about 10 mg a day and women about 18 mg. Common, inexpensive salts such as sulfates, fumarates and gluconates are good. Again, diabetics often show a problem with iron metabolism and high blood ferritin levels. This is *not* due to excessive intake of iron in their food at all, but rather the inability to excrete the iron efficiently.

Zinc is also deficient in our diets generally. Whole grains and beans again are the primary source, yet what little grains we eat are almost all refined with the nutrition removed. Eating whole grains and beans (legumes) every day will go a long way in raising your levels. The elderly, the poor, and people who drink alcohol have the lowest levels generally. The RDA is 15 mg and you have to be careful not to take too much zinc as amounts over 50 mg can cause side effects. This is a heavy metal and can accumulate in the body. The problem in diabetes is zinc *metabolism* per se rather than with deficient intake. There are many clinical studies showing poor zinc metabolism in blood sugar conditions. Common, inexpensive salts such as citrates, sulfates, or oxides are good.

Boron is acknowledged as an essential element, but the RDA has never been set. It was only in 1990 that boron was even accepted as essential! A valid estimate is 3 mg a day, but Americans generally only eat about 1 mg. Our soils are boron deficient, our food is boron deficient, and vitamin supplements rarely contain what you need. Boron is necessary for calcium absorption among many other important processes. You would think that all widely sold vitamin and mineral supplements would contain 3 mg of this inexpensive and vital element, but very few actually do. Any common salt such as citrate, or even plain boric acid is fine. It must be emphasized how important it is to get boron in your diet every day as our soils and foods are very deficient. You cannot absorb calcium without sufficient boron. Fortunately the research here is overwhelming. Get 3 mg a day of boron.

Manganese has overwhelming research on it for its value in human and animal nutrition. The RDA was only recently set at 2 mg and many people do, in fact, get that much in their food. Whole grains, beans and leafy vegetables are the best sources. We only have about 20 mg of manganese in our entire bodies. You can take any normal form such as sulfates or oxides.

Copper also has an RDA of 2 mg. Common salts such as citrates, oxides or gluconates are good. Americans only get about half this much in their food. Whole grains and beans are the best source. Some people have low copper blood levels while others have high levels. Our bodies contain a total of only about 150 mg. Anything over 15 mg daily could cause side effects as it is a heavy element, but it is almost impossible to get excessive copper in your diet even with copper water pipes in your home. Inexpensive salts such as citrates, gluconates or oxides are very bioavailable.

Silicon is an ignored element with no RDA set even though it has been proven essential in human and animal health. You will almost never find this in any vitamin supplement. A good dose is 10 mg although you probably don't need that much. It isn't toxic, so 10 mg would be a safe and effective amount. Silicon levels in common foods vary so greatly it is hard to be more precise. Plain silica gel (silicic acid) is the best form to take. Do not use supplements claiming that horsetail herb will supply this as this is not a good source - make sure the label says silicic acid. One major need for silicon (not to be confused with silicone which is a polymer of silicon and oxygen) is for bone and joint metabolism and calcium absorption. Why aren't vitamin companies putting this inexpensive, essential element in their formulas?

Iodine is most needed for thyroid metabolism. The RDA is 150 mcg and most vitamin supplements have this. There are only about 30 mg (30,000 mcg) of iodine in your body and three fourths of this is in your thyroid gland. If you have low T3 (triiodothyronine) or low T4 (L-thyroxine) you must take the bio-identical hormones, as taking iodine supplements will not raise your hormone levels. Seaweed and kelp is the best source, but the problem here is that they are *too* good! While Asians often eat sea vegetables as a staple, a mere teaspoon of kelp powder can contain twenty times the RDA and cause side effects such as skin problems. Megadoses of any mineral are clearly contraindicated.

Chromium has finally gotten an RDA of 120 mcg. This is toxic in high amounts so don't exceed 400 mcg. The research is most impressive here. Chromium has dozens of published studies showing that people with diabetes usually have deficient levels due to lack of chromium in their food. It must always be emphasized that we need *all* the known essential elements and not just ones like chromium that are proven to benefit glucose metabolism. Again, whole grains are the best source and the refined grains we eat lack any significant amounts. You can take inexpensive chelates (a metal ion bound to non-metal ions) here. Do not listen to advertising telling you that a patented form is the "best" or "only" form that works. The research on chromium and blood sugar metabolism is overwhelming. This must be in your supplement program.

Vanadium has finally been accepted as an essential element (not a mere trace element), but no RDA has been set. There is an overwhelming recent research on blood sugar metabolism for vanadium. Scientists around the world have studied this for diabetes and Syndrome X in dozens of published studies and reviews. Therefore vanadium becomes overemphasized as a diabetes mineral and the other supporting minerals that work with it are ignored. While there is no RDA, a daily dose 1,000 mcg (1 mg) is sufficient. It is not a good idea to take more than this, although *short term* studies have used more. Using more than one milligram is very irresponsible and will result in vanadium toxicity eventually. *Take 1 mg or less daily.* Inexpensive chelates or vanadyl sulfate are both good choices. You will almost never find this in vitamin supplements. This must be in your supplement program as it is proven to be essential not only for blood sugar metabolism but your general health.

Molybdenum has an official RDA of 75 mcg, but some scientists feel this is too low. You'll find this in most vitamin-mineral supplements. Inexpensive common salts are all good sources. Molybdenum is safe and non-toxic even though it is a very heavy metal. Research on molybdenum is extensive and goes back decades. Progressive farmers use this to fertilize their soils, and ranchers to insure the health of their livestock. Deficiency is not widespread here, but taking a mere 75 mcg a day is good insurance especially since dietary intake varies so greatly.

Selenium has an official RDA of 70 mcg which was only recently established. Deficiency is common because the main source is whole grains and most all our grains are heavily refined. Chelates are the best source here. Taking 200 to 400 IU of natural mixed tocopherol vitamin E works synergistically and helps selenium metabolism. Do not take more than 200 mcg as toxicity can occur over this amount. It is a heavy metal and will accumulate in the body if overdoses are used. This is a very important antioxidant element and fights free radicals. Studies have shown people with low selenium intakes have more cancer, heart and artery disease, diabetes, and other illnesses. Fortunately, many vitamin formulas contain the 70 mcg you need.

Germanium is something you almost never find in any vitamin-mineral supplement. There is no RDA here. Science has proven this is, in fact, essential and 100 *micrograms* would be a good dose as it is an ultra-trace element. In 1988 a very impressive review was published in the journal Medical Hypothesis complete with 72 references showing the importance of germanium in human and animal nutrition. Very irresponsible promoters offer 100 mg (100,000 mcg!) doses which is one thousand times what you need - a three year supply every day! Germanium sesquoxide is safe, but germanium dioxide is not. You will almost never find a supplement with 100 mcg of germanium for a complete minerals program. This is an essential element.

Strontium has no RDA, but is definitely essential and needed for calcium absorption. Do not confuse this with radioactive strontium-90! A good dose would be 1,000 mcg (1 mg) a day. A chelate or aspartate is a good choice. There is no need to take more than this although some irresponsible natural health "experts" recommend much more. Food and blood analysis studies around this world show that 1,000 mcg a day is certainly enough. It is a shame none of the supplement companies are including a necessary element like strontium in their formulas.

Nickel has no RDA, but is definitely an essential element. This is an ultra-trace element and 100 mcg would be a reasonable dosage based on various analyses of human dietary intake and blood analyses. The published research unfortunately has concentrated on animals rather than humans, and looked more at dangers and toxicity than value and necessity. The few human studies we have are most impressive however. Due to irresponsible manufacturing practices a few people have excessive levels in their bodies in certain areas where metal processing plants pollute the environment. You'll almost never find meaningful amounts in any supplements, so look for one with 100 mcg.

Tin has no RDA, but is definitely an essential element. It is also an ultra-trace element with a reasonable dosage of 100 mcg. The same comments apply regarding research on tin as to that of nickel. Human research has found low tin levels in various pathological conditions and diseases. We need more human research on tin. You'll almost never find meaningful amounts in any of the supplements currently in the marketplace.

Cobalt is a very neglected element although it is the central atom for vitamin B-12. Humans cannot synthesize B-12 without available cobalt, and vitamin B-12 supplements are barely absorbed. We probably only need about 25 mcg of cobalt a day, but it is not toxic and you could certainly take up to100 mcg. This is a very important ultra-trace element that has been completely neglected by the natural health industry. It cannot be emphasized enough that research shows how important cobalt is even though it is needed in such tiny amounts. In 2005 there is only one supplement containing cobalt in biologically meaningful amounts (from yours truly, of course.)

Cesium has no RDA, but is certainly essential. This ultra-trace element has proven value from extensive research, especially in human blood, but it is almost impossible to find in any supplements. 100 mcg would be a reasonable dose, although irresponsible promoters have been recommending much larger quantities supposedly to cure cancer and "alkalinize" the body.

Rubidium has no RDA, is not a mere trace element, and is definitely essential. 1,000 mcg (1 mg) would be a reasonable dose. Why is an element that is needed in such large amounts and found in large amounts in common foods misnamed a "trace" element and so ignored? You will not find this in any meaningful amounts in any but one supplement sold in 2005 (again, yours truly).

Let's talk about other essential and possibly essential elements. *Lithium* is definitely essential, but we seem to get sufficient amounts in our food. The idea of giving people 1,000 times the needed amount for depression is irresponsible and most dangerous. *Europium* seems to be essential, and research will probably validate this within the next ten years. *Gallium* seems to be essential, and its importance in bone metabolism has already been demonstrated. *Lanthanum* has considerable research behind it and is probably essential. *Indium* is claimed to have numerous benefits on Internet sites, but published research simply doesn't verify any of this. *Neodymium* has shown potential in animal as well as human metabolism. *Thulium* (not thallium) has soil and edible plant studies to indicate its importance, and animal studies will soon tell us more. *Praseodymium* has some animal and human research which indicates value for our health.

There is much science on using supplemental magnesium, chromium, selenium, zinc, and vanadium to treat diabetes. While this is certainly going in the right direction, the point is missed. *We need all the essential elements and not just some of them.* All elements work synergistically and harmoniously together in concert as a team. You must get *all* of them, and not just some of them. There is little point in taking just a few elements, when we know there are about twenty we need. It's just not realistic to get a blood test for twenty or more minerals. The answer obviously is just to take the ones we know we need and may be deficient in.

Since nearly all the available mineral supplements are woefully deficient what can you do? Look up "mineral supplements" on the Internet and you'll find the one that has the 20 minerals you are known to need - calcium, magnesium, iron, zinc, boron, manganese, copper, silicon, iodine, chromium, vanadium, molybdenum, selenium, germanium, strontium, nickel, tin, cobalt, cesium and rubidium. If you're not on the Internet, just go to the public library and they'll help you.

62

Chapter 10: Your Basic Hormones

Insulin is the most obvious hormone involved in glucose metabolism, but it is only one of our basic fourteen hormones. We should understand that *all hormones work together synergistically in concert together in harmony as a team.* People with blood sugar dysmetabolism have generally been shown to have other hormones out of balance. It is important that you try to balance all your basic hormones. The level you had at age 30 is the ideal; you want to strive for youthful hormone levels. You do not want "normal" levels found for older people. We will go over each one of these separately. In the next chapter we'll talk about how to test your hormones with blood and saliva.

As with minerals, all your hormones work together as a team. If one member of the team isn't doing well, all the other players are strongly affected. It is of little value to balance one or two of your hormones and ignore the others. All your basic hormones must be balanced as much as possible in order for them to work together harmoniously. Men and women have exactly the same hormones only in different amounts. Let's briefly discuss your basic fourteen hormones:

Testosterone
DHEA
Melatonin
Pregnenolone
Growth Hormone
T3
T4
Insulin
Androstenedione
Progesterone
Estradiol
Estrone
Estriol
Cortisol

Testosterone is not the "male hormone" at all, even though men have about ten times as much as women. Men and women both need youthful levels of this primary androgen. Please read my book *Testosterone Is Your Friend - A Book for Men and Women*. This is the most researched, comprehensive, and informative book available on testosterone. Men cannot have hyper levels as the testes cannot overproduce this. Even if men oversupplement with testosterone, the excess basically spills over into estradiol and estrone rather than higher testosterone. Literally over 90% of men over the age of 50 have low testosterone and would benefit from supplementation. Women have only about a tenth of the blood testosterone that men have, but they can have deficient or excessive levels. Hyper levels in women can only be lowered by diet and lifestyle, not dangerous prescription drugs. High levels of testosterone, androstenedione and DHEA in women are called "androgenicity" and are a hallmark of polycystic ovaries - a very common condition. Studies repeatedly show diabetic men generally have deficient levels, while women generally have excessive ones. Doctors generally have no idea how to accurately measure testosterone, much less administer it. They usually prescribe dangerous injections, toxic oral salts, or - at best - overpriced patches and weak gels. Transdermal creams or gels, and sublingual tablets (sublingual liquid drops taste terrible however) forms are the preferred methods. Transdermal creams and gels generally only deliver 20% into the blood. DMSO solutions deliver about 99%, are safe and effective, but are not allowed under FDA regulations. Nor are nasal sprays. Men make about 6-8 mg a day so they generally only need about a 3 mg (3,000 mcg) daily dose in their blood. This means a man would use a daily 3 mg sublingual tablet or drops and a woman would use a daily 150 mcg sublingual tablet or drops. Women make about 300 mcg a day, so about 150 mcg in their blood is a good daily dose since they store testosterone more efficiently. If a man gets a 100 g tube of 3% (3g per 100 g) cream, each half gram will have 15 mg and he can expect 3 (20%) mg to actually go into his blood. The tube will therefore last over six months (200 days). If a woman gets a 100 g tube of a mere 0.15% (150 mg per 100 g) cream each half gram will contain 750 mcg and she can expect 150 mcg (20%) to go into her blood.

Androstenedione levels generally parallel testosterone since this and androstenediol are the direct precursors to testosterone in our bodies. You generally do not have to measure this or supplement it. Taking androstenedione is not a reliable way to raise testosterone as it stops working after a period of time and then produces estradiol and estrone instead of testosterone. In some men it never works at all. If a woman has high testosterone or DHEA it would be a good idea to test her androstenedione as well. The only way to lower hyper levels in women (again, men do not have hyper levels) is by diet, exercise, and balancing the other basic hormones. Androstenedione was classified as a prescription drug in 2004 and is now a felony to possess or sell.

DHEA is the third androgen. This is very much a life extension hormone and is critical to your health and longevity. Studies again show diabetic men are usually deficient while women can go either way. Men rarely have excessive levels, while women sometimes have too much DHEA along with too much testosterone and androstenedione. As always, you are looking for the youthful level you had at age thirty. If low, women can take half tablets (12.5 mg) of DHEA orally and men can take the regular 25 mg tablets. *Never* use DHEA unless you have proven by blood or saliva analyses that you are low. This is a very powerful hormone and excessive levels are harmful. A few people will find they cannot metabolize oral DHEA and it simply raises blood estrogens (especially estradiol) instead of DHEA levels. Transdermal creams are not effective here because of the poor absorption. Injections are not practical nor natural. DMSO solutions are not FDA approved, but you can make your own. Men can use 3.0 mg a day in DMSO and women 1.5 mg a day. Do not buy "7-keto DHEA" as it is an unproven and expensive promotion.

Melatonin is a powerful *antioxidant* hormone. Melatonin is much more powerful and beneficial than the media tells you and has even been studied for cancer therapy. Even though levels fall from the time we're 18, it is essential you test your melatonin level if you are over the age of 40. You cannot assume you are low just because most older people happen to be low. Hyper levels are medically unknown (except maybe with pineal tumors). A few people are melatonin deficient throughout life and would benefit from early diagnosis. We have discussed the vital importance of antioxidants and oxidative stress in blood sugar conditions. This is a very underestimated hormone despite numerous published studies showing major benefits (including immunity enhancement and antioxidant properties) in many diseases. Taking 3 mg of oral melatonin is generally sufficient, although women may not need this much and can take a tablet, say, four or five nights a week. *Only take this at night* when our levels naturally rise and never during the day. Taking this during the day would produce negative effects. You must test melatonin at 3:00 AM with a saliva test kit.

There are literally dozens of valid animal studies proving the benefit of youthful melatonin levels for diabetes and blood sugar disorders in laboratory animals. When you have this many published studies from clinics around the world you can be sure that the human studies will be just as good. Fortunately we do have one very excellent human study on melatonin and diabetes. At Granada University in Spain (Journal of Pineal Research v.35, 2003) both blood and saliva testing showed diabetics to be about 40% lower in melatonin. Here age matched type 1 and type 2 patients of both sexes were used. Plasma melatonin averaged only 8.98 pg/ml in patients, but 14.91 in healthy controls. This is most impressive since both type 1 and 2, and both men and women patients were used. More human studies on melatonin will be forthcoming not only for diabetes, but many other illnesses.

Pregnenolone is the "orphan" hormone, like estriol, with very little research despite its great importance to our health and well being. Studies on pregnenolone and diabetes are almost nonexistent. Ironically the one available published study showed *high* pregnenolone levels in diabetics. This is the "grandmother" hormone from which all the other sex hormones are derived. Pregnenolone is *the* brain and cognition hormone, and our levels fall at about the age of thirty-five to forty and then stabilize. Despite the lack of research here you must balance your pregnenolone level so all your other hormones can work effectively. Men can take 50 mg if they prove to be low and women about 25 mg. You can get a doctor to do a blood test for this, or you can test this yourself with a saliva kit. You are looking for the youthful level you had at age thirty as always. This will help keep your mind, memory and cognition strong in your elderly years as this is the most important brain hormone of all.

Growth hormone is the most expensive hormone of all because 1) it is difficult to make such a complex molecule, and 2) the collusion between pharmaceutical companies to keep the prices high. Veterinary GH for cows and pigs is inexpensive, but no less complex or easier to produce. Just because GH is expensive does not mean it is any more important than any other hormone, or that you will get any more dramatic effects. GH metabolism is disrupted in blood sugar conditions, and patients can have low, normal or even high levels; you just cannot generalize here. Fortunately the Chinese can now produce Jintropin® for about $120 or less a month (30 IU). You need to understand that this is a tightly controlled prescription drug. Any HGH product you see sold over the counter is worthless, especially homeopathic GH and GH "secretagogues". You can legally buy this on the Internet from Mexican online pharmacies without a prescription for your own personal use. You do not need to inject this if you dissolve it in ethanol or propylene glycol and use it sublingually. You can also dissolve it in DMSO and use it transdermally (or sublingually). One mg equals 3 IU. You must remember this so you don't get confused - *one milligram equals three International Units.* The average adult needs 1 IU (0.33 mg) a day. It is very difficult to blood test GH levels, and GH rises dramatically about 1,000% (ten times) around midnight after you go to sleep. You cannot saliva test for this, and *IGF-1 levels do not parallel GH levels* despite the "conventional wisdom". Ill informed people who tell you otherwise prove their ignorance. You need to *go by actual results* here. Just go by real world results rather than blood testing. After, say, three months of use did you gain lean muscle mass and lose fat mass (you won't lose weight per se)? Did your cholesterol levels improve? Did you have more energy and just simply *feel better*? Did you find real and not just imaginary benefits? Most anyone over the age of 50 should get real world benefits.

T3 (triiodothyronine) and T4 (L-thyroxine) are your two thyroid hormones. Thyroid metabolism is generally slow in both type 1 and 2 diabetics. Get an inexpensive blood test for these. Test your FREE T3 and FREE T4, and do *not* let the doctor test the traditional TSH and T3 uptake; these do not accurately indicate thyroid function. Again, *you must test your free T3 and free T4* regardless of what your doctor tells you. Doctors know little about thyroid diagnosis and this includes endocrinologists. Here you cannot accept low normal values even though they are technically "in range". *You need average or better values.* T3 and T4 are both bioidentical hormones with no side effects whatsoever when used properly. That's right - Synthroid® and Cytomel® are exactly the same as the hormones in your body. Do not use Armour Thyroid from pigs as it contains both T3 and T4, and very few people are low in both - treat T3 and T4 separately. For people with excessive levels only diet and lifestyle will lower them; do not get surgery or irradiate your thyroid gland!

Insulin can be measured directly, and some people with blood sugar problems should measure theirs directly as part of a comprehensive diagnosis. For most people the glucose tolerance test (GTT) is much more informative as it tells the *response* of the insulin to a sugar load. The *response* of insulin is more important than the blood levels per se. The GTT test is excellent and very underused. Because of the epidemic of insulin resistance and other blood sugar conditions a GTT should be a routine part of a yearly physical rather than measuring insulin per se. This is a very accurate and inexpensive test and should be routinely done. If you have a fasting blood sugar level of 85 of less you probably don't need a GTT. Do not accept the usual figure of 100 or less as it just isn't good enough. Fasting blood sugar is a very accurate indicator, and if yours is over 85 mg/dl get a GTT test.

Progesterone is not just a "female" hormone although it derives from "pro-gestation". Women should read my book *No More Horse Estrogen!* to learn more about the benefits of progesterone. Buy a product with about 1,000 mg per two ounce jar. All women over the age of 13 should test their progesterone levels since even teenagers can be deficient. You must measure this according to your monthly cycle. After menopause it doesn't matter, of course, when you measure it. Postmenopausal women can safely use this any three weeks of the month without testing since their ovaries no longer produce this. Men can use 1/8 teaspoon five days a week directly on their scrotums to protect against excess estrogens as they age. Progesterone is therefore *anti-feminizing* in men. Men need youthful levels of progesterone just as women do. Please read my book *The Natural Prostate Cure* to learn more about why they need this.

Estradiol (E2) is the strongest, and potentially the most dangerous, of the three basic estrogens. Most American women are up to their ears in estradiol and estrone, so the idea of estrogen supplementation is generally irrational on its face. Men over 50 generally have more estradiol than their postmenopausal wives! Only diet and lifestyle will lower hyper estradiol levels, not toxic prescription drugs. Very few women will need supplementary estradiol. Low normal values are fine here since Westerners have high levels and *low normal levels are preferred.* Vegetarians and rural Asians have lower levels. Any teenage girl or young woman who has any kind of gynecological problem should test all three estrogen levels. Patches are unnecessarily expensive, oral pills are not absorbed well, transdermal creams deliver only about 20%, sublingual drops are almost unknown (but most effective), and DMSO solutions not approved by the FDA. Transdermal creams and sublingual drops can be prepared by a compounding pharmacist if you get a prescription and 50 mcg a day in the blood would be a good dose. Estradiol is very powerful and should only be used by women who are actually out of range.

Estrone (E1) is the second basic estrogen. The same information and advice equally applies as with estradiol. Estrone is not as powerful as estradiol, but is still very potent. High levels cause a wide range of health problems. For the few women who are actually low out of range in estrone they can use transdermal creams or sublingual drops just as with estradiol. Women are looking to deliver about 100 mcg a day into their blood.

Estriol (E3), like pregnenolone, is the other orphan hormone that has almost no research available especially when compared with estradiol and estrone. Common sense tells you that women must maintain youthful estriol levels. Men are rarely deficient in this. Estriol comprises about 80% of human estrogen, and is the "good" or beneficial estrogen. Doctors do not measure estriol nor prescribe it, and normal pharmacies do not carry it! Only a compounding pharmacist can supply it legally, but it is available on the Internet inexpensively. Get a 0.3% transdermal cream or gel (300 mg per 100 gram jar) and use a half gram a day. Sublingual drops in oil should contain about 500 mcg per drop. Vaginal gels are effective, but most women find them inconvenient. Never use oral tablets as they are very ineffective. If a blood or saliva test shows you are low you want to deliver about 500 mcg a day into your blood. Strive for high normal ranges here since rural Asian women and vegetarians have higher levels.

Cortisol is the stress hormone. Researchers agree that diabetics tend to have higher levels of cortisol. High levels indicate inability to deal with stress on a daily basis. The ideal way to measure this is a 24 hour, four sample diagnosis. For most people simply one test at 8:00 or 9:00 AM is sufficient. If you have high cortisol you must eat better, take supplements, balance your other hormones, *exercise*, and somehow deal with the stressful factors in your life. Only diet, exercise, and balancing your other hormones is going to lower your cortisol levels. Deficient levels are unusual.

70

Chapter 11: Hormone Testing

Currently the medical profession is in the Dark Ages when it comes to basic hormone testing. This includes endocrinologists who are *supposed* to specialize in the diagnosis and treatment of hormonal balance. Even the most prominent diabetes specialists simply have no idea that all the basic hormones should be balanced in order to successfully treat and cure blood sugar problems- their only concern is insulin. Balancing your basic hormones really can be very simple, inexpensive, and straight forward as you have already seen in the previous chapter. Fortunately, you can test most of your hormones at home with saliva test kits for about $30 apiece. Saliva testing has been used successfully for decades in clinical settings, and it is only in the last few years it has been offered to the general public. You simply send your saliva sample to a diagnostic lab for RIA (radioimmunoassay) testing. Saliva always gives free, bioavailable hormone levels and never bound, unavailable ones. You can readily find such testing services on the Internet by typing in "saliva hormone testing", "hormone testing" and similar terms on your favorite search engine.

Test your free testosterone, not your total or bound. You can do this with a saliva kit or with a blood draw. If you get a blood test you must explain to the doctor you do not want your total or bound levels tested, and you're not interested in any meaningless bound-to-free ratios. Look for the youthful level you had at the age of 30 and not the level "normal" for your age. Women must do this even though they only have one tenth the amount men do. Literally 90% of men over the age of 50 are deficient. Women can have hyper or hypo levels.

Test your DHEA or DHEA-S (sulfate) with either a saliva kit or a blood draw. Look for the youthful level you had at the age of 30. Remember that people, especially women, can suffer from hyper levels which are just as harmful as hypo levels. DHEA levels generally fall as we age, especially after the age of 40.

71

Your melatonin must be tested at 3:00 AM with a saliva kit, unless you want to pay a fortune to stay overnight in a sleep lab and get woken up at that time for a blood draw. Look for the level you had at the age of 30. Doctors have no interest in testing or prescribing melatonin since they don't understand how important it is. Also, it is sold over the counter so there is not profit in it for them. Our melatonin levels fall from the time we're 18 until they almost disappear by our seventies. Most everyone over 40 would benefit from melatonin supplementation, but don't assume you are low just because you are getting older.

Pregnenolone is the forgotten or orphan hormone, and doctors don't even know what it is or care. Yes, this includes endocrinologists generally. There is almost no research done on pregnenolone amazingly enough. Test this with a saliva kit or a blood draw. In 2005 there is only one lab offering saliva testing for this. Look for the level you had at the age of 30. Levels fall at about the age of 35-40 and then tend to stabilize. Hyper levels are rare. Again, don't assume you are low just because you are getting older. Everyone is biologically unique.

Growth hormone (GH) cannot currently be tested with saliva, and is difficult to test with a blood draw due to the fact it varies a lot during the day. The way it is measured in clinics is to take a blood draw every six hours in one day for a total of four samples. Another means is 30 minute draws for two hours for a a total of four samples. The results are then averaged out. *It is best to go by results here.* Since testing is so difficult just go the the actual real world *results* you get from supplementation. If you are over 50 the odds are your rhGH levels are low and you could benefit very much from taking it. Use 1 IU (0.33 mg) daily sublingually in DMSO and see what results you get in 90 days. You are better off just to *go by results* until saliva testing becomes available. Then you'll be able to take four saliva samples and send them into a lab.

The medical profession is really walking in darkness when it comes to thyroid testing. Doctors will usually waste your time and money testing your TSH (thyroid stimulating hormone) and T3 uptake instead of your free T3 and free T4. In 2005 there is no saliva testing offered, but this situation should change due to demand. Getting your free T3 and free T4 tested is very inexpensive and only costs about $30 each plus the office visit. Go in at about 9:00 AM fasting. Fortunately you can go to websites (like www.healthcheckusa.com) and get this done for under $100 *without a doctor*. Do *not* settle for low normal ranges here, but *look for midrange levels*. If the range is 1-10 and you are a 2 or 3 that just isn't good enough. In such a case you would need to supplement until you are at least a 5. Ranges and results differ from lab to lab; there is no universal range. 100 mcg of T4 and 25 mcg of T3 (it is always a 4:1 ratio) are good starting doses. You can get bioidential T3 (Cytomel®) and T4 (Synthroid®) legally on the Internet from Mexican online pharmacies without a prescription for your personal use under Section 21 of the U.S. Code. Do *not* use Armour® pig thyroid unless you have equally low both T3 and T4.

Rather than test your insulin per se it is better to get a glucose tolerance test (GTT). You drink a 75 gram measured cup of glucose, wait an hour and have your blood sugar level tested with a blood draw. If your insulin is effectively metabolized your blood sugar will fall back to normal. Testing plasma blood glucose per se is part of the standard blood analysis. Make sure your glucose level is 85 mg/dl or less; do not accept the "normal" limit of 100 or more.The GTT test is inexpensive, accurate, and should be done routine for anyone with symptoms of the metabolic syndrome or anyone over the age of 40. In actuality it is not commonly done at all. You must request it.

Men don't need to test androstenedione, but women should if they have either a high DHEA and/or testosterone level. All three of these hormones are "androgens" and women who have hyper levels of any or all of these suffer from such problems as polycystic ovary syndrome (PCOS). Androstenedione levels generally parallel those of testosterone.

Pre-menopausal women should test their progesterone levels with a saliva kit according to their cycle, and use transdermal progesterone if they are low. This includes teenage girls and young women. Post-menopausal women can simply use progesterone any three weeks of the calendar month since their ovaries are no longer active. Men can, and should, use small amounts of transdermal progesterone (i.e. 1/8 teaspoon five days a week), but don't need to test it.

Teenage girls, pre-menopausal and post-menopausal women should all test their estradiol, estrone and estriol levels with a saliva kit according to their cycle. Men don't need to do this unless they are using testosterone supplements (which aromatize into estradiol and estrone), or suspect any kind of hormonal imbalance such as prostate problems, gynecomastia, etc. Doctors, including endocrinologists, do not test for nor prescribe estriol, nor is it sold in normal pharmacies. Doctors blindly prescribe estradiol and estrone supplements to women without testing their levels.

Cortisol is the stress hormone and can be tested with a saliva kit. You can do this with blood about 9:00 AM fasting, or you can buy a saliva kit when you take four different saliva samples in a 24 hour period. Just taking one blood or saliva sample in the morning should be sufficient to see if you have high cortisol levels. Hypercortisol (high) is all too common in all Western societies. Only diet, exercise and lifestyle will help you lower cortisol. Hypocortisol (low) levels are uncommon, but you can take bioidentical cortisol (oral hydrocortisone) supplements if you have this problem.

Saliva hormone test kits should be sold in every pharmacy, drug store, and health food store, but surprisingly are not. You can readily find sources on the Internet under "saliva hormone test" or "saliva hormone testing" using your favorite search engine.

Chapter 12: Heart Disease and Cholesterol

We need a separate chapter on blood fats because this is one of the most important factors in blood sugar conditions and *the* most important indicator of CHD. One of the hallmarks of Syndrome X and other blood sugar conditions is high cholesterol and triglyceride levels- dyslipidemia. High *triglycerides* are more important that total cholesterol levels here. Normally you don't have to get overly involved in your HDL (high density) versus your LDL (low density) levels, but in the case of the metabolic syndrome we do. Divide your total cholesterol by your HDL level and you should get a ratio of 4.0 or less for men and 4.5 or less for women. For example, if your total cholesterol is 200 and your HDL 50 you would get 4.0 ratio. Low HDL and high LDL levels are characteristic of blood sugar conditions generally. The average adult American has an average cholesterol level of about 240, and a level of 200 is considered "good". Baloney! A good level is about 150 no matter what age, race or sex you are. Lower cholesterol levels are easily obtainable (even if you have genetically high cholesterol) by simply cutting down on meat, eggs, and poultry, and eliminating all dairy products from your diet. Even those genetically predisposed to higher levels can easily keep them under 200 by eating well, taking proven supplements, balancing your basic hormones, and getting regular exercise of some kind. Keep your triglycerides well under a 100 level. Please read my book *Lower Cholesterol Without Drugs* to see how easy it is to keep all your blood lipids at healthy levels naturally, safely, and effectively without resorting to toxic, dangerous statin drugs.

To be clear about this you must be concerned with:

TOTAL CHOLESTEROL
TRIGLYCERIDES
HIGH DENSITY CHOLESTEROL
LOW DENSITY CHOLESTEROL

Researchers around the world agree that both type 1 and 2 diabetes, insulin resistance, and impaired glucose metabolism are highly correlated with dyslipidemia. There is no reason to review this overwhelming research as the scientists of the world are in basic agreement on this issue. Our emphasis will therefore be on practical and effective ways to lower our blood fats naturally. *Diet is the most important* of course. Proven supplements, especially beta-sitosterol, flax oil, beta glucan, soy isoflavones and guggul sterones- are the second means. Natural hormone balance is the third, and regular exercise the fourth. Fasting once a week on water from dinner to dinner will also help you lower blood fats.

Supplements will only help you if you *eat well*. The most important supplement is 300 to 600 mg of beta-sitosterol. Beta-sitosterol is found in literally every vegetable you eat. The studies on lowering blood fats with beta-sitosterol go back over three decades. Most Americans only eat about 300 mg a day and vegetarians about twice that much. We eat too many omega-6 fatty acids and not enough omega-3s. Flax oil is the best known source of omega-3 fatty acids, and a better choice than fish oil for many reasons. Our food is very deficient in omega-3s, and very excessive in omega-6s. Beta glucan is the third supplement. Beta glucan is the most powerful immune enhancer known to science and that includes prescription drugs such as interferon alpha. Beta glucan has also shown effectiveness in lowering blood lipids. Please read my book *What is Beta Glucan?* to learn just how powerful and effective this really is. People of all ages will benefit from taking 200 mg of more of beta glucan a day. Isoflavones are the fourth supplement. Taking 40 mg of mixed daidzein and genistein soy isoflavones is the most practical and realistic way to get the benefits of soybeans. Western people simply don't eat enough soy foods to get sufficient isoflavones in their diet. Guggul gum is an ancient Ayurvedic remedy and taking 25 mg of guggul sterones will help lower cholesterol and triglycerides. Only use this for six to twelve months as it is "exogenous" and not found in your body or in common food. A few people are going to be biologically incompatible with guggul, so it you get any side effects just stop taking it.

People who tell you that cholesterol is not an important indicator of CHD health and longevity prove their complete lack of knowledge in this area. It has become faddish to say, "cholesterol doesn't count", so people have an excuse to continue their high fat diets. People who go even farther and tell you that low cholesterol is somehow "dangerous" are simply frauds. Some elderly people are so sickly that they lose their ability to manufacture cholesterol despite a high fat diet. Therefore their lower cholesterol levels are *not* indicitive of good health at all, but rather of morbidity. The chart below from the Multiple Risk Factor Intervention Trial (MRFIT) proves beyond any doubt that total cholesterol should ideally be about 150 mg/dl. (Archives of Internal Medicine v.148, 1998). 361,662 men from 40 different countries aged 35-57 were studied over a period of six years. The ones with low cholesterol had only 3 deaths per thousand every year, while the ones with high cholesterol had 16 deaths per thousand annually. They summarized this as, "The association between serum cholesterol and six year risk of CHD was continuous, graded and strong over the entire range…"

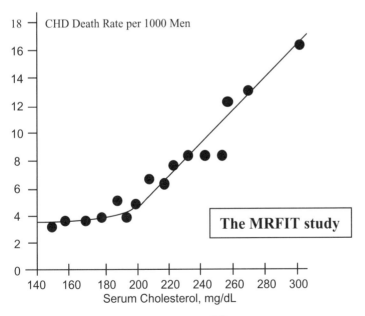

The famous Seven Countries Study has covered over 25 years. Reviewing all the known factors in coronary heart disease they concluded, "Over 50% of the variance in CHD death rates in 25 years were accounted for *by the difference in mean serum cholesterol.*" A later follow-up stated, "Across cultures, cholesterol is linerally related to CHD mortality." The American Heart Association has consistently advised that the evidence linking elevated serum cholesterol to CHD is overwhelming. The legendary Framington Heart Study found that total cholesterol, triglycerides, HDL and LDL levels taken together were *the single most important determinant* of heart disease.

Americans eat about 42% fat calories and most all of them are from saturated animal fats. Substituting vegetable oils is simply lessening the harmful effects. Canola oil is a promotional fraud (seen any canola plants lately?), despite the hype and promotion by the so-called health food industry. Olive oil is not "good for you" no matter what you read somewhere, although it is a good choice of oils. Corn, safflower, sunflower and olive oils should be used in moderation. Soy oil tastes terribly unless it is highly refined. Sesame oil is very expensive, and toasted sesame oil is a condiment. Palm and coconut oils are meant for tropical peoples living in tropical climates. You should eat less than 20% fat calories and these should be from vegetable sources as well as seafood. This is very easy to do when you're not eating red meat, poultry, eggs, dairy products, fried foods, and junk foods.

At the University of Tor Vergata in Rome (Acta Diabetologica v. 40, 2003) people with metabolic syndrome were studied. The mean triglyceride level was a whopping 193. Again, the triglyceride count is the most meaningful blood lipid figure. The mean total cholesterol was 225. Their fasting blood sugar was 108, they were overweight, had high HDL and low LDL levels, hypertension, as well as high insulin. These people were given exercise capacity tests on a treadmill. They were all found to have diminished cardiovascular capacity, which indicates a much higher likelihood of heart and artery disease. People with metabolic syndrome die earlier and have a poorer quality of life, especially due to CHD conditions of all kinds. Triglycerides are the most important lipid indicator of blood sugar problems and you must keep them under 100. Sweets of all kinds including honey and maple syrup will raise your triglycerides levels even on a low fat diet. Vegan sugar addicts will often have elevated triglyceride levels despite eating no saturated fats or animal foods at all.

Hydrogenated oils, often called trans-fatty acids or partially hydrogenated oils, are the very worst fats. These are made by taking cheap oils (such as cottonseed) and forcing hydrogen gas into them under extreme pressure and heat with a platinum catalyst. Make sure you have none of these in your house such as margarine or shortening. Margarine is not, "better than butter" at all- it is even worse.You can buy non-hydrogenated, non-dairy spreads made of coconut and palm oils as a *temporary* transition away from butter and margarine. Read the labels on any food you buy to make sure the word "hydrogenated" is not listed. Eating in fast food restaurants is almost guaranteed to get trans fats into your body. Eating in *any* restaurant is risky since the types of oils and fats used in their foods are not mentioned on the menu. Studies around the world over the past decades have proven repeatedly just how harmful these trans fats are despite their popularity.

If you are over the age of 40 you should basically be taking all the supplements listed in *Chapter 6: Supplements*. The most important cornerstone supplements are beta-sitosterol, flax oil, beta glucan, soy isoflavones, and guggul sterones (but only for about six months). There are other supplements you can take like 3 grams of guar gum, 3 grams of fruit pectin (apple or grapefruit), 1,200 mg of lecithin, 3 grams of glucomannon, and 3 grams of sodium alginate. Please do not fall for such promotional scams as policosanol, red rice yeast, "modified" fruit pectin, and overdoses of niacin. Regardless of your age you should be taking a complete mineral supplement with the 20 needed minerals in the required amounts. You can find the one formulated by your author if you simply search the Internet under "mineral supplements" as it is the only complete mineral supplement in the world with all these vital elements in the biologically required amounts clearly stated on the label.

Doctors do not understand the importance of our basic hormones on our blood lipids. If you are over 40 you definitely need to test and balance your testosterone, DHEA, progesterone, pregnenolone, and melatonin, as well as your thyroid hormones T3 and T4. Women should also test their estradiol, estrone and estriol. Please read *Chapter 10: Your Basic Hormones* for more information on this. Cholesterol itself is, in fact, a hormone and is the biological source of all our sex hormones including pregnenolone, DHEA, testosterone, androstenedione, progesterone, estradiol, estrone, and estriol. Deficient or excessive hormone levels interfere with cholesterol metabolism. Doctors have no idea that our basic hormone levels strongly affect our cholesterol and triglyceride levels, so they don't bother to test hormone levels in people with high blood fats.

In 2002 the Mississippi Regional Cancer Center published a study, "Hypercholesteremia Treatment: A New Hypothesis" (Medical Hypotheses v. 59, 2002). These progressive doctors treated people with high cholesterol and triglycerides by balancing their basic endocrine levels using bioidentical hormones. They tested their levels and then appropriately prescribed DHEA, testosterone, T3, T4, pregnenolone, progesterone, estradiol, estrone estriol and cortisone. These doctors realized that our entire endocrine system must be in balance, and all our hormones work together as a team in harmony. We need more such progressive clinicians and more such enlightening studies.

Keeping your blood fats low will go a long way to keep you healthy and live a long, enjoyable life. Heart and artery disease is the major cause of mortality and blood fats are the most accurate indicator of CHD health.

Chapter 13: Obesity

We won't spend much time demonstrating that obesity is second in importance only to diet as a factor in blood sugar problems. Everyone agrees this is true. No one disputes the influence of being overweight. *A whopping 80% of type 2 diabetics are overweight!* Half of American adults are overweight or obese, and people in other countries are quickly following our path. With affluence comes obesity and high rates of all types of disease ironically. We will therefore spend our time discussing how to realistically lose weight and stay slim.

The Department of Health and Human Services found that losing a mere 7% of body weight resulted in more than a 50% reduction in incidence of adult onset diabetes. For a 200 pound person this is a mere 14 pounds. Just a one fifteenth drop.

Being overweight has almost every negative effect on your health imaginable. Obesity is clinically associated with high insulin, high glucose, hypertension, high cholesterol, high triglycerides, increased insulin resistance, high CRP levels, high homocysteine levels, high uric acid, high leptin, and low antioxidant levels. Add to this list high cardiovascular disease rates, early death, poor quality of life, increased oxidative stress and free radicals, high cancer rates of most types, lowered immunity, increased inflammation, and higher rates of depression and other psychological problems. The only positive factor, ironically, is stronger bones due to increased body mass index.

It is only in the last two decades we have seen obesity affect American children and adolescents, especially Latins, Africans, Asians, and Amerindians. Type 1, type 2, insulin resistance, hyperinsulinemia and hypoglycemia, hypertension, high cholesterol and triglycerides, are all alarmingly increasing in these overweight children. Type 1 diabetes used to be called "childhood onset", and type 2 called "adult onset". Now children commonly are coming down with type 2 diabetes. The distinction is blurring. One important factor here is the public (which are really government schools and not "public" institutions) school lunch program. Children are fed high fat, high sugar, heavily refined foods with little nutrition. Dairy products and other food subsidy programs are promoted. Children also commonly eat meals in fast food restaurants. The food at home isn't much healthier.

The American Diabetes Association, the North American Association for the Study of Obesity, and the American Soceity for Clinical Nutrition recently issued a statement (American Journal of Clinical Nutrition v. 80, 2004) Weight Management Through Lifestyle Modification for the Prevention and Management of Type 2 Diabetes. "Overweight and obesity are important risk factors for type 2 diabetes. The marked increase in the prevalence of overweight and obesity is presumably responsible for the recent increase in type 2 diabetes. Lifestyle modification aimed at reducing energy intake and increasing physical activity is the principal therapy for overweight and obese patients with type 2 diabetes. The prevalence of diabetes in the U.S. continues to rise by epidemic proportions. This increase parallels the rising rates of obesity and overweight observed over the last decade. Indeed, as BMI increases, the risk of developing type 2 diabetes increases in a dose-dependent manner. The prevalence of type 2 diabetes in obese adults is 3-7 times that in normal weight adults, and those with a BMI greater than 35 are twenty times as likely to develop diabetes as those with a BMI between 18.5 and 24.9. In addition, weight gain during adulthood is directly correlated with an increased risk of type 2 diabetes. Obesity also complicates the management of type 2 diabetes by increasing insulin resistance and blood glucose concentrations. Obesity is an independent risk factor for dyslipidemia, hypertension, and CHD and thus, increases the risk of cardiovascular complications and cardiovascular mortality in patients with type 2 diabetes. Weight loss is an important goal for overweight and obese persons, particularly those with type 2 diabetes because it improves glycemic control. Moderate weight loss (5% of body weight) can improve insulin action, decrease fasting blood glucose concentrations, and reduce the need for diabetes medications. Moreover, improvements in fasting blood glucose are directly related to the relative amount of weight loss."

Want clinical proof from Cornell University (American Journal of Clinical Nutrition v. 46, 1987) that you can literally eat all your want and lose weight and never be hungry? Women were allowed to eat all the whole natural foods they wanted as long as they had 20% or less fat calories. *They could eat 24 hours a day!* In only 30 days they lost considerable weight by just eating foods lower in fat. The ones who ate the 30% fat diet lost no weight. Again, the average American eats about 42% fat calories and most of these are saturated animal fats. There are many more similar published clinical studies showing the very same results.

Realistically how does one lose weight, stay slim, never be hungry and enjoy your food? *Making better food choices* is the key here. Along with making better food choice there are many proven natural supplements to take that keeps your metabolism at peak potential. Natural hormone balance is basic here. Lastly, regular exercise is always a part of maintaining normal weight.

This is part of the chart from the "Calorie Density" chapter in *Zen Macrobiotics for Americans.* This is how many pounds of each of the following foods you would have to eat in order to get 2,500 calories. You could eat 0.9 pounds of peanuts or almost 12 pounds of grapes for example. To give you some idea of this:

vegetable oil 0.6	honey 1.8
butter 0.8	French fries 1.7
peanuts 0.9	potato chips 1.8
walnuts 0.9	corn chips 2.0
chocolate 1.0	turkey 2.1
beef sirloin 1.2	ham 2.1
chuck steak 1.4	lamb chops 2.2
cheese 1.5	ww pasta 3.1
white sugar 1.5	chicken 3.2

avocado 3.3	blueberries 8.8
eggs 3.4	apples 9.4
salmon 3.9	potatoes 9.6
ww bread 4.0	soymilk 10.1
navy beans 4.8	grapes 11.9
shrimp 4.8	carrots 13.0
brown rice 5.1	onions 14.8
pinto beans 5.3	oranges 15.6
sweet potato 5.4	cantaloupe 18.2
oatmeal 6.0	cauliflower 20.2
bananas 6.4	spinach 21.0
corn 6.5	green beans 21.9
mangoes 8.3	cabbage 22.8
squash 28.8	cucumbers 32.8
celery 32.8	lettuce 39.0

It's obvious that meat, poultry, eggs (50% fat calories), and dairy products are basically highest in fat and therefore highest in calories. Whole grains and beans are very filling, yet low in fat and calories. Vegetables and fruits are the lowest of all.

Please realize we only need two meals a day. The less you eat the better. Americans eat twice the calories they need. A man only needs about 1,800 calories a day, and a woman about 1,200 calories. Don't eat breakfast and you'll have more time in the morning. Or you can eat breakfast and supper and skip lunch. You'll save time, money, and energy not eating three times a day. Soon this will seem very natural to you, and you won't want to eat three meals a day anymore. You will probably not be able to fast until you are well. If you try fasting for 24 hours and feel weak or dizzy just eat something sensible like a whole grain sandwich, a hot bowl of soup, some brown rice, or similar whole complex carbohydrate dish.

You can eat all you want, never be hungry, and stay slim and trim just by choosing healthier foods to eat.

Chapter 14: Exercise is Essential

If you have most any form of cancer you can lay on your dead rear end, watch TV, rarely get any exercise at all, and still get well in a year if you do all the other things you're supposed to. This is NOT true at all with diabetes and blood sugar disorders. YOU MUST EXERCISE REGULARLY. You can do resistance or aerobic exercise, or both, but *you must exercise regularly*. There is no way around this! No matter how well you eat, how many proven supplements you take, and how well you balance your endocrine hormone system, you still need to exercise to cure diabetes and similar blood sugar conditions. The literature is overwhelmingly clear on this.

Walking is probably the best and most enjoyable single exercise of all. A simple half hour brisk walk of two miles a day is all you really need. Of course, *two* brisk half hour walks totaling four miles a day would be *twice* as good. Resistance exercise is just as good as aerobic exercise here, and the combination of BOTH resistance and aerobic would be the ideal. Tai chi just isn't realistically going to help you here as it is extremely hard to learn and doesn't get your blood flowing.

At the University of Perugia in Italy a fine article was published "Make Your Diabetic Patients Walk." It was found that the more walking the patients did the more they improved. Blood pressure fell, cholesterol and triglyceride levels fell, they lost weight, their waist measurement was smaller, and fasting glucose levels were lowered with no other lifestyle changes than merely brisk walking two or more miles a day.

At the renowned Harvard Medical School two heavily referenced reviews were done on exercise and type 2 diabetes. Regular physical exercise proved to be important in both the prevention and treatment of type 2 diabetes. Regular physical exercise with dietary restrictions increased energy expenditure which leads to decreased body weight, increased insulin sensitivity, improved long-term glycemic control and lipid profiles, lower blood pressure, and increased cardiovascular fitness.

Two very good studies were done at the University of Barcelona in Spain. Both type 1 and 2 diabetics exercised regularly for three months. Their physical fitness and aerobic capacity improved of course. Their insulin requirements were reduced, their waist measurement shrank, their blood pressure fell, Lp(a) levels fell, and their blood lipid profile improved. All this occurred with no change in diet or supplements, just regular exercise.

Diabetes is epidemic in Finland as in all European countries. At the National Public Health Institute it was shown that both resistance and aerobic exercise are effective in normalizing blood sugar metabolism in two separate studies. The role of physical activity in the prevention of NIDDM is of utmost importance. Both circuit-type resistance training and aerobic endurance exercise had beneficial effects in subjects with impaired glucose tolerance. The University of Kuopio and Helsinki University found the same effects with type 1 diabetics.

It is difficult to treat obese diabetics for many reasons. However, overweight women at the University of Texas performed regular exercise. Exercise training resulted in significant weight loss and lowered the insulin response to an oral glucose load (i.e. improved insulin sensitivity). Remember this was done with no change in diet. Exercise alone results in meaningful weight loss. If the women had been given a low fat, whole grain based diet, and a full spectrum of supplements and minerals they would have further improved insulin response and lost even more weight.

At the University of Vienna in Austria men with long-term type 1 diabetes exercised regularly for four months. Their oxygen uptake increased and their insulin requirements decreased. Physical exercise training in patients with type 1 diabetes mellitus improved metabolic control and various aspects of health related quality of life. Besides enhanced cardiorespiratory capacity, this is an important subjective benefit in patients with longstanding insulin dependent (type 1) diabetes.

Postmenopausal women, especially obese ones, in America can be difficult to treat because they usually have multiple health conditions. At the University of Maryland in Baltimore obese postmenopausal women aged 50 to 65 performed resistance training (RT) exercise regularly for a few months. The gained strength, lost weight, lowered their body fat per cent, and improved their insulin sensitivity. The conclusion was that RT has the potential to ameliorate and perhaps prevent the development of insulin resistance and may reduce the risk for glucose intolerance and NIDDM in postmenopausal women. Just simple exercise accomplished this.

At Maastricht University in the Netherlands a review with a full 130 references was published. They found physical training played an important, if not essential role in the treatment and prevention of insulin sensitivity.

At Aichi Medical University in Japan a mere 30 minutes of low intensity bicycle exercise in obese diabetics (the hardest to treat), significantly enhanced the lower level of insulin-induced glucose uptake. Also another study at Aichi type 1 diabetics simply walked every day and improved their glycemic control.

At Kansai-Denryoku Hospital in Japan two separate studies of type 2 diabetics were done. In the first study only exercise was used. Their insulin sensitivity immediately improved, and their glucose and triglyceride levels both fell strongly. The researchers felt the lower trigylceride levels were the most important factor for the improvement of diabetes with exercise. In the second study exercise was combined with a low-fat traditional Japanese-style diet. They concluded that short-term (7 days) low-intensity physical exercise combined with traditional diet reduced serum triglycerides, insulin resistance, and fasting glucose levels. Only one week of exercise accomplished medical miracles.

At Syracuse University two separate studies using resistance rather than aerobic exercise were done. In the first study resistance exercise reduced glucose levels in type 2 female diabetics. They found resistance exercise offered an alternative to aerobic exercise for improving glucose control in diabetic patients. To realize optimal glucose control benefits, you must follow a regular schedule that includes daily exercise. In the second study male and female diabetics got the same results from exercising with no other treatments or lifestyle changes.

At Robert Wood Johnson Hospital in New Jersey a review with 69 references was published. Both type 1 and 2 diabetics lowered their blood pressure, lost weight, and lowered their cholesterol, as well as improved glucose and insulin parameters with minimal regular exercise of any kind.

Researchers at the University of Western Australia did four studies and used resistance (strength training) exercise just 30 minutes a day, three times a week- 90 minutes a week- and found this provided a practical addition to lifestyle management of type 2 diabetes in only eight weeks. Resistance exercise (circuit training) was found to be an effective method that improved functional capacity, lean body mass, strength, and glycemic control of patients. One of the studies found that moderate exercise and a diet (including fish) high in omega-3 fatty acids improved various diagnostic factors for type 2 diabetes. Another study lowered glucose 13% and insulin 20% just with mild exercise. At St. Vincent's Hosptial in Sydney type 1 diabetics improved their health with just 45 minutes of cycling a day. Again, feeding whole complex carbohydrates prior to exercise prevented hypoglycemia.

At the University of Copenhagen strength training for 30 minutes just three times a week showed dramatic improvement in type 2 diabetics. Insulin sensitivity increased markedly in only six weeks. In a second study strength training again for just 30 minutes a day three times a week improved various test measurements of blood sugar metabolism. *Just 90 minutes a week is all you need.*

At Saint-Louis Hospital in Paris the researchers found physical exercise to be essential in the treatment of type 2 diabetes. Their extensive review left no doubts about this. In another study there men were given eight weeks of endurance exercise just 45 minutes a day twice a week which resulted in a marked increase in insulin sensitivity among other important benefits such as less body fat and more muscle mass. To show how simple and easy this can be, older women were simply asked to walk more each day for eight weeks with no change in diet or other factors The women did not have to take time to specifically go for walks, but simply walked more during each day. They found improved glucose tolerance and a reduction in systolic and diastolic blood pressure in overweight women at risk for type 2 diabetes. This demonstrated that activity can be accumulated throughout the day and does not have to result in weight loss to benefit such a population.

Exercise training is associated with improved insulin sensitivity found the doctors at the University of South Carolina. Both vigorous and non-vigorous exercise resulted in improved insulin sensitivity in men 40-69 years of age.

At the famous Brigham & Women's Hospital in Boston a massive 26 page review was done with 168 references on exercise in both type 1 and 2 diabetes. There is no doubt that regular exercise has numerous benefits for blood sugar conditions. Physical exercise is an important adjunct in the treatment of both NIDDM and IDDM. There is now extensive epidemiological evidence demonstrating that long-term physical exercise can significantly reduce the risk of developing NIDDM. Glucose uptake, glucose control, insulin sensitivity, GLUT4 (a marker for glucose uptake) is raised, and glucose transport are all improved. This is the most extensive published review ever done.

At Nagoya University in Japan three heavily referenced

separate reviews were done showing that regular exercise not only improves glucose metabolism in diabetes, but also in other lifestyle-related diseases. Insulin sensitivity also strongly influences cardiovascular health including hypertension, ischemic coronary disease, and blood lipids. They found evidence to support the theory that, combined with other forms of therapy, mild exercise training increase insulin action. Along with evident benefits in health promotion, moderate-intensity exercise plays an important role in facilitating treatment of various diseases. It is well established that patients with impaired glucose tolerance are characterized by sedentary lifestyles coupled with poor physical fitness and insulin resistance. They also pointed out if diet therapy is not followed, good control of blood glucose will not be achieved.

Royal Victoria Hospital in Canada published a review "Intense Exercise has Unique Effects on Both Insulin Releases and its Roles in Glucoregulation." This showed overwhelming evidence that exercise helps regulate glucose utilization and production.

At RMIT University in Australia one study and two reviews were done. Aerobic exercise training was found to be a potent and effective primary intervention strategy in the prevention and treatment of individuals with insulin resistance.

People of African, Asian, Amerindian, and Latino origin are much more susceptible to diabetes genetically. Research at Texas Women's University compared Mexican women with non-Hispanic women. Here they got even *better* results lowering insulin and blood sugar from merely walking 50 minutes a day.

The University of Waterloo in Canada did one study, Exercise Improves Glucose Tolerance, and one review with a full 75 references. 1 in 20 Canadians are outright diabetic with many more having various forms of blood sugar dysmetabolism. The University of Alberta found pregnant women with gestational diabetes responded very well to resistance (strength) training.

At the CERAMM in France a review with 132 references was published. They found exercise can improve many of these abnormalities, and the mechanisms underlying exercise-induced benefits were clarified during the past decades.

Female diabetics in Greece were exercised at the University of Thrace and got many benefits in just four weeks. A combined training program of strength and aerobic exercise induced positive adaptations on glucose control, insulin action, muscular strength and exercise tolerance in women with type 2 diabetes.

Type 1 diabetes can have trouble with vigorous or extended exercise due to hypoglycemia. At the University of Udine in Italy this was solved by giving moderate exercise for an entire hour at a time with whole grain snacks. They suggest feeding complex carbohydrates before exercising to keep blood sugar levels up.

People of all ages with blood sugar problems benefit from exercise of any kind. Young men with hypertension exercised regularly at the University of Ulleval in Norway and improved their insulin sensitivity, which also lowered their blood pressure.

The Japanese now suffer from far more diabetes as they Westernize their diet and lead sedentary lifestyles in the cities. Osaka University did three excellent studies showing insulin sensitivity, plasma glucose, insulin levels, weight, body fat and the HbA1c blood marker are all improved dramatically by short-term moderate exercise such as simply walking every day.

Researchers in Poland at the Medical Academy found tumor necrosis factor (a blood marker) to indicate insulin sensitivity. (Low TNF is good.) They discovered regular physical exercise decreases TNF system activity, and that decrease may be responsible for the concurrent increase in insulin sensitivity.

91

In just 10 days glucose intolerant men strongly improved their status with just moderate exercise for just 40 minutes a day at the University of South Florida. Moderate, short-term exercise was effective in improving glucose tolerance and insulin response. Now imagine what you can do with just walking every day year after year.

Type 1 diabetics at Vanderbilt University got immediate results from either low or moderate intensity exercise. Repeated episodes of prolonged exercise of both low and moderate intensities blunted key autonomic and metabolic counter-regulatory responses to next-day hypoglycemia in type 1 dia-betes. Type 1 is harder to deal with due to lack of pancreas activity.

Overweight men and women pre-diabetics at the University of Pittsburg (average age only 39) were given moderate exercise along with a lower calorie diet for 16 weeks with impressive results. Exercise combined with weight loss enhanced post-absorptive fat oxidation, which appears to be a key aspect of the improvement in insulin sensitivity in obesity.

At East Carolina University in North Carolina otherwise *healthy* overweight subjects were found to be insulin resistant and therefore pre-diabetic. Here their total daily physical activity was taken into account and not just formal exercise. Their physical activity encompassed a wide range of intensity and volume which minimizes the insulin resistance that develops with a sedentary lifestyle.

When you have blood sugar dysmetabolism of any kind you must get regular exercise. Ideally you will do both resistance and aerobic, but it just doesn't matter as long you do one or the other. Walking is the easiest to do and most relaxing. You'll live longer and live better by merely taking a brisk half hour walk every day.

Other Books from Safe Goods Publishing

Testosterone Is Your Friend – Roger Mason	$ 8.95 US
	$14.95 CN
The Natural Prostate Cure – Roger Mason	$ 6.95 US
	$10.95 CN
No More Horse Estrogen! – Roger Mason	$ 7.95 US
	$11.95 CN
Lower Cholesterol Without Drugs – Roger Mason	$ 6.95 US
	$10.95 CN
What Is Beta Glucan? – Roger Mason	$ 4.95 US
	$ 6.95 CN
The Minerals You Need – Roger Mason	$ 4.95 US
	$ 6.95 CN
Zen Macrobiotics for Americans – Roger Mason	$ 7.95 US
	$11.95 CN
Lower Blood Pressure Without Drugs (Fall 2006) – Roger Mason	
The ADD and ADHD Diet	$ 9.95 US
	$14.95 CN
ADD, The Natural Approach	$ 4.95 US
	$ 6.95 CN
Eye Care Naturally	$ 8.95 US
	$12.95 CN
Cancer Disarmed Expanded	$ 7.95 US
	$11.95 CN
Overcoming Senior Moments	$ 7.95 US
	$11.95 CN
The Secrets of Staying Young	$ 9.95 US
	$14.95 CN
Atlantis Today- The USA	$ 9.95 US
	$14.95 CN
2012 Airborne Prophecy	$16.95 US
	$24.95 CN
Analyzing Sports Drinks	$ 4.95 US
	$ 6.95 CN

For a complete listing of books visit our website:
www.safegoodspub.com to order or call (888) 628-8731
For a free catalog call (888) NATURE-1